When Life Gives You Lemons

A Collection of Reader-Submitted Medical Stories

Kerry Hamm

Copyright © 2019
Kerry Hamm
All Rights Reserved.

Disclaimer:

Names, locations, and portions of the details included in this book have been altered to protect the privacy of those involved.

<u>Warning:</u>

This edition features light profanity that may be offensive to some readers. The profanity has been used sparingly and in each instance the usage was included in the submission. I have chosen to leave some of these words in to emphasize portions of the stories.

By now, I am sure you are all too familiar with my *Real Stories from a Small-Town ER* series, which were collections of stories told to you from my time as a registration clerk in Ohio. If you are new here, don't fret! You don't have to worry about a 'certain order' for *any* of my books, including this one!

I have since moved on from the hospital scene, but that hasn't stopped readers from submitting stories of their own experiences from the medical field. Over time, I have received hundreds of stories-some funny, some sad, some downright scary or grotesque-and have worked with my readers to bring these stories to you in a follow up to my last *Real Stories* volume.

If I've learned anything from writing my series and compiling this book, it's that none of us are alone. We're all proof that we've seen some seriously messed up things out there, right? We have seen the good. We've seen the bad. We've seen the downright vile and disgusting. And then, we've seen the humor in these situations and we've been fortunate enough to share them with one another. There is a certain peace in knowing that as no matter how crazy we feel, we have formed solidarity amongst ourselves, knowing that for every bad day you've had, others have had them too. We have worked through the challenges of getting up and facing another drug seeker, another child abuse case, another young death, and another 'how the heck did that even happen?' moment together. You guys are not alone, and this book reaffirms that.

Several of the stories have been edited to bring you clear-cut and clean versions of tales submitted by loyal readers. I have done my very best to edit out hospital and town names, and in some cases my submitters wished to withhold their initials and other details from publication or requested that I edit stories for grammar/spelling. Some stories have been edited for length. I do my very best to preserve a reader's humor and emotions, as well as capture the reader's personality when I edit these submissions. To be clear, I do my best to remove ANY identifying information from these submissions, and sometimes that may include altering specific stand-out details with the submitter's permission. This is to prevent readers from searching for patients online, thus revealing the identities of parties involved. This is done carefully, and I work with readers to keep touchy submissions as close to the initial submission as possible.

Though some of the stories in this collection are horrifying, I am glad none of us are alone in what we've witnessed or experienced.

Cheat Sheet

Some readers have been confused about terms used in this series. Here's a quick list to help you out!

LEO: Law Enforcement Officer

ETOH: shorthand for Ethyl Alcohol or Ethanol; commonly used to describe intoxicated individuals

Bus/Rig/Truck: Ambulance

M.D.: Medical Doctor

R.N.: Registered Nurse

MVA: Motor Vehicle Accident

EMS: Emergency Medical Services

EMT: Emergency Medical Technician

PD/FD: Police Department/Fire Department

D.A.: District Attorney

BOLO: Be on (the) Lookout

DCFS/CPS: Department of Children and Family Services/Child Protective Services

SNF: Skilled Nursing Facility. This can be a nursing home or one of many facilities for patients in need of supervised care

AMA: Against Medical Advice

LWBS/LBT: Left Without Being Seen/Left Before Triage

LOL: Little Old Lady

You spoke. I listened. You may notice formatting changes in this edition. There are details in the section 'A Message to Readers.'

It Seemed Like a Good Idea at the Time

My husband had just been released from the hospital following a very serious illness. He was quite weak and wobbly, but really wanted a shower. The Occupational Therapist recommended that we get a bath chair to set in the bathtub. That way, he could just sit as he showered. Well, I had a better idea: (Insert Redneck Alert here). He could just use one of our lawn chairs! You know, the ubiquitous white plastic chairs with decorative slits in the back and seat?

So, okay, we got off to a good start. He was thoroughly enjoying a shower after his long hospital ordeal.

I started to dry him off with a towel. I asked him if he could stand up. He said, "I think I'm stuck."

Me: "What do you mean you're stuck?"

Him: "Well, my testicle is stuck."

Me: "Stuck where?"

Him: "In the chair."

Me: "Well how did that happen?"

Him: "It slid through one of the slits in the seat."

Me: "We'll, okay let me think."

That's how I stalled for time. I crawled into the bathtub behind him and looked under the chair to verify the situation. Yup, that was indeed the problem.

So, Manipulate. Testicles are squishy, right? I decided to try to squeeze it back through the slit. That didn't work and husband expressed some major discomfort!

Next idea was Refrigerate. Testicles shrink, right? I put some ice in a washcloth and applied that. More discomfort, but no progress.

Okay, let's Lubricate. I sprayed PAM on the situation. Again, no progress, but much discomfort expressed!

I told husband that I would have to call 911.

I hadn't given much thought to what I would say....

"911, what's your emergency?"

"Uh, I need help to get my husband out of the bathtub."

"Did he fall?"

"Uh, no. He's just stuck."

"He's stuck how?"

"Uhh... Well... Okay....he has his testicle stuck in a lawn chair."

"His testicle is stuck in a lawn chair?"

"Well, yes."

"Ambulance is on the way."

"Thank you."

I do want to say that the 911 dispatcher, the ambulance crew, and the firefighters were the consummate professionals on this call.

And thank heavens the firemen had a reciprocating saw...

-A.H.

Illinois

Bright Idea

When a father and son approached the registration desk, I could immediately tell who the patient was. The son was in his late teens. He was sweating bullets and was on the verge of tears. His father had a smirk stretched across his face as he elbowed his son in the small of his back and urged, "Well, get on up there and tell her what you did."

The patient leaned in and whispered to me, "I, uh, need to see a doctor."

After I gathered the patient's name and date of birth, I asked for his chief complaint.

"I, uh," he stammered.

"He had a bright idea," his dad said with a hearty laugh. He was so amused with his own joke that he had to step back for a few seconds before he could compose himself.

The patient was obviously afraid to share his chief complaint. Truthfully, I was becoming frustrated because I was technically on break. My supervisor was hired straight from the pits of hell, so no matter what, your 'break' starts at a set time and ends at a set time. I had already missed 10 minutes of my 30-minute lunch, and I was starting to think that I wouldn't get a break at all.

"What," I asked harshly, before realizing I was losing my temper and reeling it back in, "seems to be the problem today?"

"Son, just tell her," the patient's father sighed.

"I, uh," the patient stammered.

Dad gently pushed the patient to the side and said to me, "He has a light bulb stuck up his ass."

Dad then went on to make a series of jokes that included, "I'm gonna light your ass up—Oh wait, you already did that," "Enlighten me as to why you'd do this," and, "Watts the matter, boy? Lighten up!"

I could have lost my job for laughing, so I bit my tongue—hard—until triage came for the patient. As soon as he was out of sight and out of earshot (so I thought), I laughed. The patient's dad peeked his head around the corner, winked, and said, "I knew I wasn't the only one who thinks I'm hilarious."

I sat in the nurse break room and ate a pack of peanut butter crackers because some jerk had found and eaten my (labeled and dated) homemade chicken salad sandwich, carrot sticks, and peach cobbler. I couldn't even watch TV on my break because a few days earlier, two nurses thought it would be a good idea to play tennis in the break room with some equipment a patient left behind, and they shattered the TV screen. They were written up. Some days, I feel like I work for a circus, not a hospital.

A few minutes after I got back from break, my light bulb patient was leaving. He was carrying a transparent Ziploc sample bag. His father made him come over to the registration desk to show me the bulb. The bag contained a plastic light bulb used for crafts. It was shaped like a traditional light bulb and was the same size as a traditional light bulb. The patient didn't say much, but I really didn't expect him to. His father said, "Yeah, the doc saw the light at the end of the tunnel and just pulled it right out with some tong things."

As the two were leaving, the father looked back and called out to me, "You've been great. Thanks a watt for your help."

I lost it and started laughing so hard that I snorted. I wish I could track down that father and talk to him about a stand-up comedy career. I don't think I've ever seen anything funnier in this job.

-D.K.
Oklahoma

Smile!

I worked in a nursing home and one of our residents was a sweet lady, but she had dementia and was a klepto. If anything was missing, we knew whose room to check. The facility had 2 units separated by the dining room and as I walked through the dining room one morning, I saw the patient sitting with her daughter. The daughter didn't believe her mother had dementia and I could tell she was angry when she motioned me over to their table.

As soon as I approached them, she started screaming about how incompetent we all were and, "Who would possibly have done this to [her] mother?!", and she "should transfer [her] mother to a different facility immediately."

I looked at her mother and she was looking up at me with a big toothy grin on her face. She obviously had stolen a much larger patient's dentures and stuffed them in her mouth. I almost choked, I was trying so hard not to laugh, and told her I would have a nursing assistant find her mother's dentures. I couldn't get away from them fast enough!

-L.B.
Florida

Happy Holidays

I was having Christmas dinner with my parents, who resided in a SNF. Sitting in a wheelchair near our table was an old lady, swaddled head to toe in multicolored crocheted afghans. I would guess her age at around 140. She hadn't said a word or opened her eyes since we had been there.

A well-dressed man in suit and tie walked by her and said, "Merry Christmas Edith!"

She showed no response at all to his greeting.

After he continued on down the hall, she popped her head out of her cocoon and said to us, "Did you hear that? That son of a bitch thinks it's Christmas!"

We laughed so hard that we probably should have been thrown out of the dining room.

-A.H.
Illinois

One Man's Emergency is Another Man's WTF

I was wheeling a discharged patient to the foyer one night, when I saw an SUV come flying through the parking lot. I assumed the driver was drunk or bleeding to death because the SUV was zig-zagging all over the place and damn near took out a row of parked cars. Finally, it came to a screeching stop just outside the ED lobby.

"They're certainly in a hurry," the LOL I was escorting out commented. She worriedly said, "I hope they're okay."

The driver of the SUV didn't even kill the engine. He came rushing out of the vehicle and practically mowed my patient and me down as he rushed to the center of the lobby and screamed, "I need help!"

I know it's not right to profile patients, but when you've been in the ED for 24 years like I have been, it becomes easier to guess why someone's in your hospital. This gentleman was young, either still in high school or was barely in college, screaming in a hospital lobby like a banshee at 03:30. I couldn't help it. My brain just screamed, "Overdose!"

My patient's husband pulled their car directly behind the SUV, but I did not feel that I could let the young man in the lobby scream incoherently at the registrar. I asked my patient if it would be okay to check on the man in the lobby. She urged me to go.

"Calm down," I said. "Tell me what's wrong."

He pointed to his SUV and stammered, "He- He- He-."

The young man couldn't finish his sentence.

"Did he take something?" I asked, as I rushed to the wheelchair corral.

The frantic man nodded.

"Jane," I said to the registrar, "call Charge and tell him I need a bed open right now."

My veins were pumping with adrenaline and so much so that I still can't remember how I got from the lobby to the SUV. I do recall that the young man from the lobby did not immediately follow me outside. I remember opening the passenger door of the SUV, but nobody was in the front seat. I don't remember what I said, but it was enough that another young man asked from the back seat, "Sir? Sir? Are you still there? I need help!"

"What did you take?" I questioned.

"Huh? Nothing!"

This man started sobbing and said, "Please don't take me to jail! I have practice on Monday!"

I noticed he was slurring his words, and I could detect what I can only tell you smelled like cinnamon alcohol and vomit. I have never been a drinker, so I don't think I could pick out Jack Daniels from Jose Cuervo. I am, however, schooled in the many types of vomit there are out there. This was distinctly alcohol vomit.

My LOL's husband hobbled over and asked if I needed help. I really didn't know how to respond to him because I still didn't know what was going on. He leaned against his walker and waited with me.

"Did you get him out?" the first male asked me, as he ran out to his SUV.

I was still standing at the front passenger door. At this point, I imagine that I looked like a deer in headlights.

"John?" asked the backseat male. "John, am I getting arrested? Is that a cop? Did you tell him I smoke crack? Why would you do that to me? I thought we were bros!"

I still don't understand what cocaine had to do with it, as neither young man admitted to doing the drug. I imagine this was a joke between the two or drunk rambling.

The first male yanked open the back-passenger door and said to me, "Hurry up! My mom's gonna kill me if we don't help him."

When I got to that door and looked inside the vehicle, I didn't know how to react. I've seen many things in my career, but this was a first.

The young man in the back seat somehow had his head stuck between the leather cushions that made up the middle bench. One of his arms was twisted in a seat belt. He was also not wearing pants or boxers. He was, however, wearing a tee shirt, socks, and sneakers. There was vomit oozing from the space in which he was stuck.

An orderly and two of my fellow (female) RNs rushed outside, all under the impression that we were dealing with a drug overdose. We tried to pry the young man out from between the seats, but he squealed during our attempts. He said something about his ear was stuck on something. We had to call a maintenance worker, who came down and removed part of the seat so we could free the young man. He had continued to vomit the entire time, so he was covered in his own sick.

Meanwhile, the driver complained and panicked over the vehicle's condition because the SUV belonged to his mother, who'd let him borrow it after he lied and stated he was going on a date. Rather than go on a date, he met his buddy at a party and they both admitted to having a few drinks. He started vomiting in the parking lot when we told him we would call the police if he tried to drive off the lot while intoxicated.

"My mom's gonna kill me," he cried. "I was supposed to be home, like, five hours ago."

That's when we learned the young men were between the ages of 15 and 17.

As soon as we freed him, backseat boy sobbed because he was afraid that he was going to get kicked off the basketball team. He also cried because the female RNs who'd helped free him saw his flaccid penis…and then he cried even harder when the same two female RNs also saw his *erect* penis. Staff had to explain to the young man that it was completely natural for this to occur, but I think he was so drunk and embarrassed that nothing we said to soothe him really mattered.

We called both boys' mothers, and both mothers requested we admit the boys 'to make sure they were okay.' We registered them as ED patients with moms' consents, and then we basically let them rest and get it all out. Both young men were fine in the medical sense. Their mothers arrived around the same time and I don't think I've ever heard more shouting in our ED than I heard that night.

-G.P.
Ohio

Grinning

I was a biology major in college, working as what would now be called a tech, at a very small community hospital during the summer. Each tech had a choice of ER, OB, or Laundry (I SAID it was a VERY small hospital). I didn't want anything to do with OB, fearing that I would break a newborn, but ER sounded good.

One evening a good-looking young guy came into our ER with lacerations from a motorcycle accident. We were busy, as always, so I was instructed to get him ready for the doctor to suture him up.

Okay, he had blood on his long-sleeved shirt and blood on his jeans, so I helped him remove his shirt. And then I asked him to remove his jeans. He just grinned at me and complied. He had neither wounds nor underwear under those jeans. I can still see his grin to this day.

-A.H.
Illinois

A.H. from Illinois also writes:

I was a Registered Dietitian working in a community hospital. I received an order to see a pt. who wasn't eating well. She was a sweet, spry 90 yr. old.

Our cooks (truly unsung heroes), would try their very best to meet a patient's request. (Including eggplant parmigiana on Christmas Eve one time).

So, I explained to the LOL that she could eat whatever looked good to her.

She replied "Honey, I'm blind."

Woops!

Listen to Your Gut

A story in your last book hit a little close to home. The story was about an officer who was playing a shooting game and had his fellow officers called on him.

My husband and I live in the only "bad" part of our small town. A few months ago, we got some new neighbors: a state police officer and a stay-at home-wife. My husband and I were happy that our street would get safer with a patrol car parked outside. I usually work nights so am often up for a few hours once I get home to relax and unwind.

Sometimes I'd hear the neighbor screaming profanities loudly and creatively. I figured what I was hearing were video games because I usually heard simulated gunfire and stuff along with it. This morning was different though, because their dogs were going crazy and would not stop barking. I also heard a person crying. I decided to call the police just in case. They were a nice couple and kept to themselves pretty well. Occasionally they had a few friends over but nothing crazy.

Later at work, I heard that the neighbor's wife had some fractured ribs and some lacerations to her face and arms, as well as a lot of bruising. So, I just wanted to let people know that it is okay to call the police and if your gut tells you something is off, listen to it!

-E.W.
Location withheld at request

Oh, Baby

My partner and I were dispatched in the middle of the night to transport a patient who said she was in active labor. When we arrived, she was lying on her porch, dressed only in a nightgown, and she was screaming. My partner left the back doors open, and when I panicked and shouted, "Holy crap, I can see the baby," he came running.

It was my first 'baby call,' so my partner and I had to make a decision. He could either let me drive and we could get to the ER (which was 20 minutes away) in about five minutes, which would likely include me clearing a bunch of trees and plowing down a few cows along the way…Or he could get us to the ER in one piece and I would stay in the back with our patient.

We loaded the patient and I kneeled at her side as she nearly tore my hand off and screamed bloody murder. She refused to let me move to check her or the baby, and she refused pain management. I believe her exact words, edited so I don't scare off your readers with the obscene number of profanities, were, "I'll tell you if the baby comes out, you son of a bitch."

After about five minutes, I saw a black-gray blur in my peripheral vision. I glanced over and saw a fat raccoon sitting in the corner of the ambulance. Just as my patient screamed, so did I.

My patient grabbed my shirt and demanded, "Why are you screaming?"

I was in total shock as I stuttered through, "There's a raccoon in here!"

The patient continued screaming and squirming, and she was squeezing my hands so hard that I couldn't feel them.

I was panicking and spouting off that I had heard that raccoons carry rabies. The animal stared at me with hatred in its eyes and stepped in my direction a few times. I think it was trying to threaten me.

My patient saw that I was focused on the raccoon and said, "Stop staring at it. Just let it stand there."

"I don't want to get rabies!" I shouted.

She yelled back, "You're going to get my foot up your ass if you don't stop freaking out!"

I took her advice and started trying to work with her on breathing techniques. She then screamed, "Just look at the [effing] raccoon! God, you're just like my husband!"

She started sobbing, but that only lasted a few seconds. Then, she was right back to screaming.

The animal in the corner knew I was scared, and it found its happiness from witnessing my fear. It teased me by standing on its back legs and wiggled its tiny little front paws. I'm pretty sure it was saying, "Fight me, bitch."

When it started approaching me, I shrieked like I'd seen a ghost and tried to run away. My patient grabbed my utility belt and hung on for dear life.

I accidentally dragged my patient off the gurney.

My patient stood up and started beating the crap out of me with my own clipboard, before the pain caught up with her and she had to lie down again. She dropped the clipboard to the floor, and my pen went rolling over to the doors.

This damn demon raccoon saw this, scampered over to the doors, and picked up my pen. This is when crap got real. You don't ever mess with a medic's pen. You just don't. That was *my* pen. It wasn't the one that I handed to patients. It wasn't one I let my partner use. That was *my* pen, and this 20-something-pound animal had snatched it up from the floor and was just sitting there, basking over the beauty of the pen's stainless-steel barrel. The animal removed figured out that it could press the end of the pen, so it did, and then it inspected the pen's medium nib.

I puffed out my chest and bowed my arms and I walked right up to that animal, shouting, "Give me my pen, you [lots of profanity]."

It wasn't afraid. In fact, it snapped at me, which sent me running back to my patient.

We rolled right up to the ER entrance, completely skipping the bay. We didn't have time to wait for the bay doors to open or time to badge through three sets of doors, just for a nurse to argue with us about the patient's condition. I mean, at this point, it was clear the baby was almost out. The patient was in immense pain and seemed to have gotten through the 'be there for me' stage. She was now in the 'give me drugs and get this thing out of me' stage. And if the raccoon didn't kill me, my patient would.

As soon as we opened the doors, the raccoon gave me a look that said, "So long, sucker," and it jumped out of the ambulance like it had just completed a heist and was leaping out of an airplane with its parachute. You can just picture two medics trying to unload a crying, screaming patient, with one of the medics shouting curses at a pen-snatching raccoon that was darting through a full parking lot.

We got the patient up to OB, and I let my partner deal with all the paperwork. I hurried back down to the parking lot and walked the entire lot at least three times, hoping the raccoon dropped my pen. I never did find it.

We heard the patient delivered about fifteen minutes after we arrived at the hospital. I wasn't surprised at all by that. I am still surprised that she refused treatment during transport. But we also heard that the patient's husband was on a business trip and the patient requested a male nurse to hold her hand during delivery. I think she was more concerned with emotional support during her labor than she was with the physical aspect. She was one tough cookie, that's all I can say.

I've since bought another pen. I now wear this one on a lanyard that I keep around my neck or in my front pocket. I'm still miffed about losing my old pen. We shared a lot of special moments. I can't even see a raccoon on TV without cussing.

   -J.F.
   Virginia

Flipping Out

I have been a nurse for 35 years; 11 of those years working in OB/GYN. I've got a host of eye rolling stories as well, but thought I'd share my daughter's story with you this time.

My daughter is an RN in the ED of a large pediatric hospital. She tells the story of her most trying, frustrating and anger-inducing parent (not patient) she has encountered in her almost 3 years on the job.

One evening, a mother and her 9-year-old daughter arrived via EMS from south of the city. In doing so, they bypassed a different campus of this same hospital, because, "they're not nice there."

The chief complaint? The morbidly obese 9-year-old had stepped on a rock… three days ago! She was complaining that her foot still hurt and that she could barely walk on it. Most of the walking difficulty was most likely due to the fact that the child weighed 68 kilos (roughly 149 pounds). After x-rays determined that there was no bone or soft tissue damage, the patient was given a prescription for crutches.

Unfortunately, the ED had had a rash of leg injuries and were out of the medium- height crutches, thus the prescription. When told this, the mom became verbally abusive and began shouting at my daughter, asking her, "How am I supposed to get those?! I don't have any transportation. We came by ambulance. You need to call Medicaid and get them to come and pick us up! And what about some pain medication, my baby is in pain!"

My daughter informed her that they were also sending the child home with a prescription for ibuprofen. Yes, that went over well...Not!

The mom then started yelling that the Medicaid van would have to stop by a 24- hour pharmacy on the way home so that they could get the prescriptions filled. (It was now nearing midnight.) At this point, my daughter left the room for fear she would say something most inappropriate to the mom. The on-duty social worker was able to arrange a ride home for the pair, but when mom was told that it would be 2 hours before their ride would be there and that they were not allowed to stop anywhere on the trip home, mom became even more irate and started cussing out everyone in her vicinity. This was all done in front of her 9-year-old, an ED full of patients and parents, as well as staff.

At this point, the charge nurse had security escort the two outside to await their ride. This was the closest my daughter ever came to cussing out a parent of one of her patients. Regardless of this type of (thankfully) rare behavior, she absolutely loves her job!

-M.G.
Georgia

Hypocrisy

M y 450-pound patient (who was already demanding EMS take him/her to get fast food following discharge) requested another physician in a profanity-laced tirade.

He/she said to me, "I'm not taking advice from a so-called doctor who doesn't take care of himself."

When I asked the patient to be elaborate on that, he/she motioned to my head and stated, "You're going bald. You shouldn't be working in medicine if you can't take care of yourself."

I generally do not judge my patients, and I usually don't let my temper get the best of me, but this left me feeling so heated that I had to leave the room before I told the patient *exactly* what I thought on the topic of self-care.

-Y.W., M.D.
Iowa

Gobble, Gobble

When my partner and I arrived on scene for possible injuries sustained in an MVA, our patient was screaming at the responding LEO. We knew the LEO was a rookie, and though we hadn't worked with him tons, what interactions we had had with him left us confused and/or angry. He wasn't the sharpest tool in the shed.

We approached the scene and intervened before the patient could get himself in trouble with the law.

"Calm down," I said. "Just calm down."

"Well!" the patient exclaimed. "How do you expect me to be calm when this jackass is asking me stupid questions like that?"

"I'm just doing my job, sir," the officer said with a sigh.

"It was a turkey!" the patient shouted back.

"Hey," I said again, "just calm down."

The patient complained, "But he's asking me stupid questions!"

"What'd he ask you?" my partner questioned.

The patient exclaimed, "He asked me to describe the turkey that I hit."

My partner and I both just kind of looked over to the LEO, who asked innocently, "What? I'm supposed to get descriptions."

"It was a TURKEY!" the patient shouted. "I don't know how to describe it. It was big and had feathers, and it looked like a turkey! I'm sure it went, 'Gobble, gobble,' as it kamikaze-ran in front of my car!"

He pointed to the woods and continued, "It ran off that way after I hit it. Do you want to put out an all-points? Start a search and rescue party? See if he has insurance, will 'ya? Oh, but that's why he ran off, I bet. He's probably uninsured."

The officer became angry and started shouting at the patient. We had to keep the two separated.

The patient refused medical treatment, but we stayed behind to act as mediators until the LEO left the scene.

-R.P.

Location withheld at request

One of our residents has a bad habit, so we put bed alarms on his cot.

Poor 90-something-year-old John sleepwalks.

That probably wouldn't be so terrible, but John also urinates on things when he's sleepwalking.

Once, he wandered into the hall and urinated on an empty wheelchair.

The last straw was when he somehow wandered to the commons, lifted the top to the vinyl player, and urinated inside.

In John's defense, he 'put the seat down' by closing the lid again.

When John's alarms go off, we're right there to help him to the restroom or back to bed.

-L.S.
U.K.

Untitled

A coworker and I were wheeling a flirtatious patient to recovery following surgery. He was loopy from the anesthesia, and he kept hitting on me, a continuation of how he behaved prior to his procedure. He was quite vulgar as he explained how he would 'satisfy' me, should I agree to a date with him. I kind of laughed it off and told him, "I don't think my boyfriend would be okay with me seeing other people."

The patient started crying and made some comment about wanting to have sex with me. I ignored the comment, and we got him settled in his room. My coworker joked about the situation, but then we just kind of went on with our shift.

I didn't think much of it because my patients say all kinds of crazy stuff when they're coming off anesthesia. I thought that since he'd been flirting with me prior to his procedure, maybe his brain just ran with it and he couldn't control it. People say all kinds of nutty things when they're coming down. I once had a middle-aged man tell me he wanted to be a gold-star gymnast. I had told him, "Good for you. Don't give up on your dreams." He cried and thanked me for my support while his wife recorded him with her cell phone.

Well, I went back to the room some time later, and the patient did not seem under the effects any longer. He did, however, seem to remember that I had confirmed my sexual status, and he was just as crude and pushy about it. I told him I was uncomfortable with him hitting on me, and I told him that if he did not stop, I would request that I not be assigned to him any longer.

The patient grabbed my crotch and tried to kiss me. I slapped his hand away from my groin and tried to leave the room, but he got out of bed and assaulted me, both physically and sexually. He covered my mouth so that I could not scream, and he stuck his hand down my pants after he pushed me against the bed. I tried to fight him off. He tore my scrubs and punched me in the back of the head. As soon as I got him off me, *he* started screaming for help and demanded to speak to my supervisor. I was in tears when I left the room because I was so embarrassed and scared about everything: having to explain the situation to anyone, feeling violated…everything.

We had to get the House Supervisor involved, and because of the severity of the accusations against me, the police were called. I tried to defend myself by showing the officers my torn scrubs. The patient had told the officers involved that he tore my scrubs when he was fighting *me* off, and he showed my superiors and the officers a bruise on his face and scratches on his arms from where I'd defended myself. But he said he wanted to press charges, so I was arrested, based purely on the patient's accusations. Screw a nurse's rights when something like this happens. I suddenly seemed to have no rights. What the patient said was enough for the officers. My boyfriend had to leave work early, take money out of our savings, and bail me out of jail. He didn't believe that I'd done anything wrong. Someone from the hospital told me that I would not be allowed to return to work until an investigation had been completed into the sexual assault claims and overall situation. The patient alleged that I had hit on him, made him uncomfortable by asking him for sex, threatened him, and that I had sexually assaulted him. I had to submit multiple reports, and everyone who'd interacted with the patient or had witnessed his behavior towards me had to also submit reports. The hospital set me up with a team of attorneys, so that was a blessing because I couldn't afford that kind of team on my own.

A hospital panel and officers conducted a thorough investigation of the history of my employment and the allegations against me, but they found nothing to suggest that I had ever been involved in the type of behaviors the patient accused me of doing. That's because I don't behave that way. My boyfriend and I are committed to one another, and not only would I never cheat, but if I *did* cheat, I would not make unwanted advances on someone. I would certainly never attempt to force myself on someone.

I was cleared of all charges after the patient admitted that he lied. He admitted to physically and sexually assaulting me. He was charged with falsifying a report and a few other things, but nothing really stuck. He couldn't be charged with rape because there was no penetration, and I was told that his actions were considered either misdemeanor or lower-level felony crimes, so that's why nothing really happened to him. It left me feeling angry and broken.

I've heard a lot of my female coworkers complaining about sexual harassment and have witnessed my coworkers being grabbed and cat-called. But I never thought it would happen to me, especially to the point that my superiors and law enforcement would be involved.

I have a lot of respect for my female coworkers for dealing with this. I'm the first male I know of that this has happened to on at a job—any job, not just healthcare. I was so shaken up that the hospital said they wanted me to go to counseling for a while. My counselor referred me to an online message board for male victims of sexual assault. I somehow found myself lost online and found support groups for male and female assault victims. I had no idea how prevalent this was for both sexes.

I just want women to know that this kind of stuff happens to men, too, and I want men to know that it's okay to talk about it. Nobody should be afraid to say no, and you shouldn't have to fight off advances from someone.

My boyfriend and I are now engaged. Everything at work has mostly gone back to normal, except that I was promoted, which isn't a bad thing. I briefly considered starting my own support group for victims of sexual and physical assault in the workplace, but I don't feel that I'm qualified. I think it's something I want to explore.

-Initials and location withheld at request

Last winter, a woman called 911 because her dog's tongue got stuck to ice in a pool from which he was trying to drink. She called back almost immediately after ending the first call, just to tell us the dog had either pulled himself loose or had salivated and loosened his tongue.

Strangest call of my career with the fire department.

-B.B.
Tennessee

My driver hit an unavoidable pot hole while we were transporting, and I'm pretty sure I had an out of body experience. My body was knocked to the floor, but my soul was hovering at the ceiling, screaming, "Why won't someone fix these roads?!"

Fix your roads, y'all. We don't have the luxury of going around when traffic won't get out of our way.

-F.R.
Indiana

A woman came to us (bondsman shop) to bond her boyfriend out of jail, but we declined the agreement for reasons I can't disclose.

Upset at our decision, the woman caused a scene. We called the police. She continued to disrupt business. We finally moved her out of the shop, but she continued harassing innocent civilians passing on the sidewalk.

The woman attempted to kick our window out. Technically, she did break the glass, but the entire window did not shatter. Her foot was stuck in the hole in the glass.

She tried with all her might to pull away as the blare of sirens neared, but this resulted in her falling backwards.

Officers found her lying on the sidewalk, with her foot stuck in our window.

-J.M.
Location withheld at request

Blemish

T.B. in North Carolina listened to this conversation between a patient and Triage in the wee hours of the morning:

Triage: So, it looks like you're in here for a strange blemish on your arm?

Patient: Yeah.

Triage: When did you notice it?

Patient: I've had it all my life.

Triage: Does it itch, hurt, or have you noticed that it's changed in color or size?

Patient: Nope. It's just a weird red thing on my arm. Wanna see?

Triage: Sure.

Patient: See? It's just a weird spot on my skin. My mom said I've had it since I was born.

Triage: Sir, that looks like a birthmark.

Diagnosis at discharge: It was a harmless birthmark.

I went to an elderly man's room one morning, woke him up, and said, "Here's your Synthroid pill."

His eyes almost bugged out of his head and he screamed, "Cyanide pill?"

Luckily, no one else heard him. They would have thought I was one of those nurses who murders their patients!

-Another gem from L.B. in Florida

Dispatch is for the Birds

A.K., a new reader from Indiana, said, "I stumbled upon your latest book and rolled my eyes at the submission about the elderly woman calling 911 for frogs in her yard. That sounded fabricated to me. I thought, 'Nobody would do that. Ever.' Well, a few days later, I was stuck answering our 911 calls. I wanted to share a call with you."

Me: 911, please state your emergency.

Caller (a female, who sounded in her 30s or 40s): I think something bad is about to happen.

Me: Just stay calm for me. Can you give me your location?

Caller: ABC Lane.

Me: What's happening right now? Are you or others in danger?

Caller: What? I don't know. That's why I'm calling you.

Me: Ma'am, I'm not sure I understand your complaint. Are you in danger?

Caller: I think so. I saw this documentary that said animals know when stuff is gonna happen.

Me: Ma'am?

Caller: What?

Me: Are you experiencing an emergency?

Caller: That's what I'm trying to tell you. I think something bad is about to happen. I think there's gonna be an earthquake or something. We're on a major fault, you know. When it happens, we're probably all gonna die. So, you might want to get some people ready.

Me: Uh... Ma'am, would you like an ambulance or medical transport to the emergency room to speak to someone?

Caller: No! I'm just trying to tell you about the birds.

Me: What about the birds?

Caller: They're flying. And there are a lot of them. Like hundreds of them. They're everywhere. And they're loud. It sounds like they're screaming, like they're trying to warn people.

Me: You're calling because you think the birds know something humans don't?

Caller: Yes! Jeeze, took you long enough to understand.

Me: You think the birds know something because they are flying in large flocks?

Caller: Yeah. You might want to tell the fire department and stuff.

Me: Ma'am, it's January.

Caller: So? Earthquakes can happen in January.

Me: But—.

Caller: I think they're doing this because something is gonna happen.

Me: Ma'am, I think they're just migrating.

Caller: Well, will you take my information?

Me: Ma'am?

Caller: Well, if you find out something is happening, you can call me and let me know. Because if I'm wrong, then I'm just gonna go watch TV.

A.K. says he took the caller's information to keep the line clear, but he never had to call her back because there never was a disaster in the area.

My guys and I pulled our patrol vehicles to the side of the road, turned on our hazards, and waited for additional patrol to arrive so we could begin setting up our DUI checkpoint for the evening.

We were parked for a mere 30 seconds before a vehicle crossed the median and slammed into both patrol cars.

The driver was heavily intoxicated.

My partner said to me, "See? I told you I shouldn't have to work overtime this weekend; they're coming to us on their own."

Easiest arrest of the night, but it set us back a bit because we had to wait for towing before we could continue with our checkpoint setup.

-G.H.
West Virginia

Break Time

A construction crew had been working just outside our ES, so there were barrels, concrete blocks, and big wooden spools everywhere. Of course, they can't work overnight—and our town is blessed to have a low crime rate—so the crew leaves everything uncovered until they can come back for the next day's work.

We'd been having a crappy night. We lost two patients to drug overdoses, and we lost another patient to an unrelated accident. On top of losing three patients, we'd seen just about every B.S. excuse to get narcotics, and then we had to call in Social Services for suspected child abuse. Like I said, it was a rough night.

Around 03:00, a medic returned. He had forgotten a signature for his paperwork.

"You know," he said to me, "that thing out front looks like a lazy Susan. You can run on it and everything. We were just doing it."

I walked outside with him and saw a large wooden circle teetering on some construction materials. It was perfectly balanced, so that someone could run on the circle and it would spin and wobble, almost like one of those rides you see when the carnivals come to town.

I, an intellectual, gathered a few of my fellow nurses (and one doctor) in the lot. We, all licensed professionals with degrees from prestigious higher-level universities, climbed up on the circle. We started by moving slowly in the same direction, careful not to tip the circle too far in one direction. We quickly noticed that even jumping did not seem to affect the balance, though.

"What are you guys doing?" laughed our Nursing Supervisor as she stood at the ES entrance.

We told her we needed to take a break, so she joined us.

So, five RNs, the Nursing Supervisor, and one doctor came up with this idea to blow off some steam by chasing each other around. We were running as quickly as we could, and the circle was rotating and wobbling so fast that I felt dizzy.

Without so much as a moment's notice, the wooden circle must have come unbalanced, because everyone went flying. It happened so quickly that I don't remember thinking much at the time. I landed near a bush. My elbow was a little scraped, and my scrubs were muddy, but I was fine.

Some of my coworkers were not so lucky.

We had to register our doctor as a patient because he broke his arm. Two of our RNs suffered from ankle injuries. Another RN hit her head and complained of severe pain, so she had to register as well. Our Nursing Supervisor had it the worst, in my opinion. She somehow landed on a board that had a bunch of nails it it…She landed so hard on that board that it was stuck to her back. She had nine nails driven in her body from her shoulder to her buttocks.

We screwed ourselves into being short-staffed because our little 'break time' cost us three RNs, our Nursing Supervisor, and our only doctor. We had to 'borrow' the ICU physicians until additional ES staff arrived.

Oh, we were punished, yes indeedy! It served us right, I believe, but the punishment was a harsh one.

My coworkers recovered just fine, but you can believe we won't be doing that again. Okay, let's get real. We probably *would* do it again, just slower or with not so many of us up there at one time. It was fun while it lasted.

-L.O.

Michigan

My first-trimester patient forgot something in our office, so I hurried outside, hoping to catch her before she left the lot.

"Oh, honey," I said as I was handing her property back, "smoking's not so good for the baby."

She snapped at me and said, "What difference does it make? I'm gonna smoke when it's born, so it better get used to it now."

She then called me a name I refuse to repeat.

I guess it's my own fault for trying to help.

-T.L.
Oregon

88 M.P.H.

The greatest call of my career happened a couple of decades ago. I don't think I'll live to see anything funnier.

Our station is in a rural community. The town is big enough to have its own police department, fire department, and hospital, but otherwise, we have a post office and a few small grocery stores. If you want to go to Wal Mart, you hop in your car and drive for about 35 minutes. All the towns surrounding us are even smaller than ours, and they're all at least 15 minutes away.

My partner was an idiot and was talking crap about his ex-girlfriend (who just also happened to be our dispatcher) on a hot mic, so it was no surprise that we'd gotten our fifth or so call in such a short span. We were supposed to go back out to boonies and transport a male who was either an ETOH patient or needed a mental health eval. I say 'back to the boonies' because we'd been out there twice already—once for a complaint of dehydration or something, and a second time because this guy stabbed himself in the hand when he was trying to skin a squirrel. You're probably asking yourself what the hell was going on, so I'll explain.

Over in one of the smaller towns, there was a kind of historical festival going on. People were dressed in old-time garb. It was much like one of your readers talked about in the submission where the idiots were kicked by the horse. These people also had horses there, and they spent a week 'roughing' it. They used outhouses, bathed in the river (some people brought camp showers, but they were discouraged from using them), hunted/fished their food, and basically pretended they were back in the early colonial days.

When we arrived, parked, and entered the main village area (a grassy area lined with vendor huts constructed out of tent poles, mud, and hay), it immediately became clear who our patient was. I mean, yeah, it *could* have been the guy who was drinking (what I'm guessing was) homemade moonshine out of a tin measuring cup, but we were *pretty sure* it was actually the scrawny guy in his twenties, who was naked and cracking a horse whip at these men and women dressed up like they were Paul Revere and Betsy Ross. It appeared he'd already gotten a few of them because a guy was over by the leatherworker's hut, blowing on a welt on his arm. His wig was hanging half off his head.

We should have waited for officers, but dispatch told us en route that they were called, so it was going to take another 15 minutes for someone to get out there. We thought that between the two of us and 20+ historical actors and visitors, we could manage to get this guy pinned and eventually restrained.

A bunch of people were trying to reason with the guy, but he just wasn't having it. When we walked up and he saw us, though, his entire demeanor changed.

He screamed, "Oh thank God! You're from my time!"

Then he looked frightened and asked, "Oh, man. But what if you're not? Are you really from the future? What year is it where you're from? Are you travelers, too?"

I told the man 'my year,' and he started sobbing. He dropped the whip, sat on the ground with his balls in the grass, and cried like a baby.

I couldn't detect alcohol on his breath as we moved in, but it was clear he was mentally unstable and was displaying signs of psychosis. His pupils were also dilated, so we were operating on the belief that he took drugs.

The patient flipped out just as we thought we'd convinced him to walk to the ambulance. He pointed to a tattoo that became visible when my sleeve rolled up, and he started screaming about how the historical actors were going to burn us alive for being witches. We couldn't physically get him under control, so he ran over to the blacksmith hut, grabbed an iron from the fire, and he branded himself on the chest with a poker. We still don't know why he did that. The blacksmith and others tried to wrestle the iron away from the patient, but even though he was clearly experiencing immense pain, he fought everyone. He managed to clip one woman on the cheek with the iron, so everyone rushed over to make sure she was okay.

We only managed to grab the patient because he tripped over someone's sneakers. Thank goodness for that person's historical inaccuracy. (Way to go, Carl.)

A few actors pinned the patient to the ground while we grabbed the stretcher from the ambulance. Of course, restraints were the next step.

On the way to the ambulance, the patient screamed about time travel. He freaked out again once we got him loaded up. He was screaming about how he was 'catapulting through time' and he didn't know where he was going to end up.

The patient's friends showed up at our station a few hours later, asking if we had the guy's MP3 player by any chance. We told them that we did not have the patient's belongings. They told us that the patient had informed them that he was going to go out in the woods to 'hang out' and try the hallucinogenic mushrooms they had obtained from an online merchant. The patient never returned to their apartment, so they thought something may have happened to him. They called the hospital, learned he was there, and then were told to check with us to see if we had the patient's belongings. They were arguing about his MP3 player when they left.

I never did much more than smoke pot when I was the patient's age, so after seeing his reaction to mushrooms, I was feeling fairly grateful. I don't think I was ever high enough to think I was a time traveler.

I *still* will sometimes be lying in bed or sitting in church and think about how high the patient must have been to 1.) strip naked in the woods, 2.) walk out of said woods and think he'd time traveled. I'll be in a meeting and think about the patient's grandkids asking, "Grandpa, how'd you get that mark on your chest?" and burst out laughing because that's gotta be one hell of a story to explain. I laugh at inappropriate times and usually can't stop laughing once I've started thinking about the guy. It's gotten me in trouble a few times, but oh well.

-H.K.
North Carolina

Weird Remedies

First responders share stories of unconventional remedies patients have attempted:

We got called to a call for a severe burn. When we arrived, the patient called to us from upstairs.

We found this patient, a male between the age of 40-60, naked in a bathtub filled with black water.

He stated he'd heard soaking in water filled with teabags helped sunburn, so he thought it would also work on his legs, which he'd burned when he accidentally set himself on fire after throwing gasoline on his backyard bonfire.

The patient stated he didn't have teabags, so he thought instant coffee would probably help, too.

He still had pieces of his jeans fused to his legs when we transported him.

-C.H.

South Carolina

Our patient sliced his thigh open while working with a chainsaw. When we arrived on scene, there was flour and blood all over the kitchen floor.

The patient's wife thought that she could use flour to create clotting.

The method didn't work so well.

-M.C.
Missouri

I had to ask for a reassignment once and only once in my ED career. A patient had come in with 'foot pain.' When she took off her house shoes, I vomited.

The patient had stepped on the plug to her vacuum and instead of seeking treatment, she'd alternated soaking her foot in olive oil and melted butter. She said she'd read somewhere that the oil and salt were supposed to accelerate healing and kill bacteria.

I was almost seven months pregnant and couldn't handle the smell or the appearance of her foot. I don't even know what happened with the patient because I became sick when anyone even mentioned her, and I had to excuse myself from the conversation.

-H.I.

Virginia

One of our frequents called our Unit Clerk one afternoon and asked if she needed to be seen for the ingestion of bleach.

We put the frequent in contact with the Poison Control Center, but she came in by ambulance a short time after.

The patient stated she felt a headache coming on, so she thought that she could prevent it by swishing a mouthful of bleach. She ended up swallowing most of the bleach.

Still don't know what the patient's reasoning was. Don't really want to know.

-N.F.

Florida

My patient checked in with two pieces of soggy French toast wrapped around his sprained ankle.

He said his grandma made him to it because it was supposed to 'absorb the pain.'

I asked the patient if this worked.

He screamed, "No!"

-K.L., M.D.
New York

Years ago, I was out on the first date with my (now) husband. I didn't have friends outside of EMS, nursing school, and other healthcare professionals, so I remember being super nervous that I was going to bring up something disgusting at dinner, just because I was so used to talking about that kind of stuff with my friends.

My date's eyes got really big just as I was about to bite into my corn dog (we went to a fair and were eating at picnic tables), so I thought I was doing something wrong.

He leaned across the table and told me to look behind me.

When I turned my head, I saw this older couple passing a can of WD-40 back and forth. They were spraying it on their joints.

What made this worse is that they spotted me and struck up conversation.

I knew the couple from EMS. They said their knees hurt from walking around the park, so they frequently used WD-40 as relief.

I told this story to my Charge the other day, and she said she's heard of patients doing the same thing. I have no clue if it works or not (and do not recommend anyone trying it), but Charge said some patients swear by it. She was serious, and I know the couple years ago weren't kidding.

-I.N.

Oklahoma

Let Me Sing You the Song of My People

At the time, I worked as a clerk in a fast-pace, high-traffic registration unit of the hospital. My coworkers and I registered patients for bloodwork, surgery, consults, and the like. We also took orders from other departments, so OB would call and tell us to enter a newborn in the system, or we'd mark a patient as expired if we received a call from any department. We were often short-staffed, and we didn't get breaks.

My boss…Oh, man. Imagine the most callus, hateful, bitter four-letter B word in history. Now triple it. This woman was a walking, talking nightmare. I think she only had a job because she screwed up our department so badly that nobody wanted to transfer over to take her place if H.R. finally let her go. This lady constantly screamed at us in front of patients, scolded patients for everything under the sun, and she would regularly tell other departments that we would take on their paperwork, which all had to be separated, Xeroxed, and assembled in a packet. She didn't care if that was too much work. Why would she care? It's not like she ever did any of it. She was such a lazy boss that she'd pass *her* work to us. If we refused to do it, she'd find a reason to fire us, or she'd find ways to punish us, like purposely underscheduling.

While we were conducting a mandatory emergency drill and could not register patients, one of my coworkers started talking about how he wanted to send his wife one of those singing telegrams. If you're not familiar with that, it's where you can hire someone to deliver flowers and sing a short song. We all started talking about our opinions on the matter, and we somehow flipped it around to answer, "Would you be comfortable if someone sent you a singing telegram at work?"

I casually stated that my ex had sent me a singing telegram once, and that I hated it and hated him for sending it.

My boss walked by and made a comment that was something along the lines of, "That's probably why you're single. How could you think someone would want you, anyway?"

I was fuming because my ex sent me that singing telegram (when I worked in another department) following a fight we had where I'd accused him of cheating. (In my defense, I found a bra behind my sofa, and it wasn't my bra.) He paid someone an undisclosed amount of money to sing to me in front of a waiting room full of patients that he wanted to break up. And, oh yes, he had been cheating on me with a woman I'd considered one of my best girlfriends. One of the lines of the song basically said he'd been using me for money and that he'd emptied our joint checking account (he did, by the way, and I never got a dime back). When I got home that day, he'd taken *everything*—even items that didn't belong to him. I was young and dumb and that moment will always remain as an emotional scar.

That was the last straw with that monster manager. I stayed until the end of my shift, but I didn't stay a second longer. Instead, I went home and searched through the phone book (gives you an idea of how long ago this was) for singing telegrams.

The next day, I clocked in as normal. My boss was on everyone's asses that morning. She was practically breathing fire down my neck. I knew I had to keep my cool for just a little while longer.

At noon, a man dressed in a heart costume walked through the doors carrying red balloons. He stopped in the lobby, pulled a piece of paper from his pocket, and then asked loudly in a sing-song voice, "Does anyone know where to find Jane Smith?"

My coworker called my boss and told her someone was out front with a delivery. She came walking out of her office with an expression that teetered between annoyed and confused.

This heart-dressed man sang the chorus to 'Take This Job and Shove It' to my boss, and then he handed her the balloons. She threw them. The balloons' strings were tied to a deflated balloon filled with sand, so they kind of landed a few feet away and just swayed in the breeze coming from the ventilation system.

My boss started stomping around our work area, screaming for someone to tell us who sent the telegram. She was threatening us and was knocking papers and file trays to the floor. I calmly put my coat on, grabbed my purse, and as I was walking by her, I shrugged and said, "I quit."

It was a risky move. Looking back, it was the most immature thing I think I'd ever done in my life. Honestly, though, I don't regret it at all!

My leaving set off a domino effect, so over the next month, that woman had to hire and train six new employees.

My daughter was hired to that department about a year ago. Since it had been some time, of course, my previous manager was no longer employed at the hospital. I mentioned to my daughter that I worked in that hospital before she was born, but I never really told her which department, and we didn't talk about it much because I'd gone on to pursue a degree in Accounting.

My daughter called me maybe a week after she'd started her new job, and we talked for a good while before I asked her how the job was coming along. She said it was busy, but she liked it otherwise.

I'm not entirely sure how we even got on the subject, but my daughter said to me, "Some old lady who works in patient escort was telling me about how this one registrar went crazy and hired someone to sing to the boss and say that they quit. She said I should be glad that the department isn't run by the same person."

My daughter laughed and asked, "Who'd even do something like that?"

I chuckled and said, "Gee, honey, I really don't know."

I still haven't 'fessed up to my daughter. I don't know if I should laugh that someone remembered what I did and continues to pass their knowledge of a clever resignation, or if I should be embarrassed. I honestly can't believe that 20-something years later that anyone would even recall that, but my daughter said someone doing something like that is "legendary."

I guess I'm legendary. Huh.

-H.P.
New Jersey

L.J., M.D. is new to the series. He writes:

I read a story regarding a woman who placed a 'healing stone' in her vagina. I can confirm this *does* occur.

Some time ago, a mother brought in a toddler for a complaint of fussiness and a rash. Nursing staff found a 'healing' salt stone in the child's pull-up.

The child was found to have a critical illness.

I'm not knocking holistic medicine as a whole, but there are some cases where I believe it's just not gonna work. This was one of those cases.

Retirement

I worked on Hospice for 12 years before I went to the ED for 27 years. Prior to those jobs, I worked in an SNF, so I've pretty much spent my entire life in healthcare. I mean this almost literally because my mother was a nurse and my father a veterinarian. I spent most of my childhood learning suture techniques, helping birth calves, and learned how to administer vaccinations before I could ride a bike. If I'd done any of that while being raised in today's society, I'm sure my parents would have been contacted by social services.

When I began in the ED, I worked days. That didn't last long. For most of my 27 years, I worked the night shift. My husband usually worked EMS on nights, so it worked for us.

I will spare you the monotonous stories from my years in the ED. Just know that I could send you many submissions that would knock your socks off. For every outrageous story, I could tell you ten about how our nights were boring. Regardless, I was ecstatic for retirement.

My coworkers threw me a party in true ED fashion. Everyone brought in an item for a carry-in, and then we became so busy that by the time we made it to the break room, other departments had come and eaten all our food. I ended up getting the only slice left from a sheet cake. I couldn't bring myself to finish it because I started crying and couldn't stop. My coworkers tried to cheer me up by saying we'd still get together for brunch and 'see' one another on social media, but I knew it wouldn't truly be the same.

Morning came, and we all rushed out of the ED like we were a herd of stampeding buffalo. My husband and I were both exhausted when we were back at home, but we decided to celebrate 'the first day of the rest of my days off' by watching the next episode of America's Got Talent that we'd recorded with our DVR. My husband even surprised me by bringing home breakfast from my favorite local restaurant.

We went to bed as normal. Hours later, I remember hearing our scanner going off in the kitchen, and my husband's cell phone started ringing endlessly. He was called in for an emergency. I fell back asleep.

When I woke up, I panicked because my alarm hadn't gone off. I hurried to feed the pets, shower, put my face on, and do my hair. I realized I didn't have enough time to make dinner, and we were running low on groceries because I'd planned on going to the market over the weekend, so I decided to stop for KFC instead. I found myself growing irritated at the girl at the window because my order was taking forever. I knew it wasn't her fault, and I was appreciative that she'd taken care to give me a fresh meal, but I was still irked.

As soon as I received my order, I raced across town and hurried inside. I tried to use my badge at the timeclock but kept getting an error message, which left me even more irritated because I knew how much of a pain in the keister is was to have our supervisor change our time.

You're following the story correctly. On my first day of retirement, I went to work out of habit. When I walked to the back and sat down at my empty station, everyone gave me a look like I'd come back from the grave. Nobody said anything, though.

It took me nearly 10 minutes to realize that I shouldn't have been there, and I only figured it out when I was asking around for my assignments and was waiting for report. My former coworkers gave me so much grief that all I could do was laugh with them.

My husband was getting out of the shower just as I returned home. He said, "You look nice."

Then he noticed I was wearing scrubs and he started laughing.

I'm secretly hoping he does the same when he retires soon, but he jokingly tells me that he wouldn't do something like that because his noggin runs properly.

On a positive note, I had the opportunity to feel the rush of being late for work one last time. And, if we're being truthful, I do kind of miss that feeling at times.

-D.H.
Washington

Super Trouble

My wife is one of the medics who sent you a message regarding the Super Bowl. She neglected to tell you that the patient she transported via private vehicle was her stupid husband. Now that we're out of the ER and resting at home, I'll tell you what happened.

When the Rams missed a field goal, I lost my temper and grabbed the nearest item to throw at the wall. That item was my wife's weighted medicine ball. It broke a lamp, bounced off the wall, and hit me in the back as I'd turned around to complain about the game. I fell, caught my ear on the corner of the coffee table, jammed the neck of my beer bottle into my eye, and ended up in the ER for a total of nine sutures.

I am 'grounded' from watching sports until I replace the lamp and get the smell of beer out of the carpet.

-Anonymous at request

Small Peanuts

I work at a long-term facility for adult patients with disabilities. My patient was involved in an MVA when he/she was younger and suffered from a traumatic brain injury. He/she has difficulties with speech. He/she will often get 'stuck on' a word and often repeat a single word or phrase. This can last 30 minutes, or it can go on for two days.

My patient's latest word was 'peanuts.'

Well, after nine hours of listening to that word being spoken by someone with a speech impediment, I clocked out and went to Dairy Queen. I'd promised my kids ice cream for their A and B report cards.

I approached the register and said to the teenaged boy at the counter, "I'd like two penis buster parfaits."

The young man turned vermillion. What's worse is that I didn't immediately realize I'd said what I'd been hearing all day. As soon as I did realize, I apologized a billion times.

The woman training the young man brushed it off and said, "It's okay. People come in here and give us crap all the time, so it's better for him to learn how to handle it now."

I tried to explain my blunder, but I think the cashiers thought I was just being a troublesome customer.

When I got back out to my car, I started laughing so hard that I had to just sit there for a few minutes before I could drive.

-A.K.
Indiana

This is Why We Can't Have Nice Things

L.S. (who's asked for her location to be withheld) writes:

I am not big on football or any sporting event. None of my coworkers are really into sports, either. So, in the middle of my shift, when I heard shouting coming from the lobby and waiting area, it didn't click in my head, "Oh duh, it's the Super Bowl."

Our registration clerk said he'd tell the person in the waiting room to settle down, and then we heard the shouting stop. We just assumed that was the end of it.

I had a 'mishap' with a young patient, so I had to go change out of my scrubs. I had toddler vomit down the front of my scrubs as I walked down the main hall to get to the ED locker room.

Right at that moment, someone in the waiting area began to shout again. I glanced over and saw a man lift one of the waiting area chairs over his head. He was swearing and shouting up a storm as he repeatedly beat the television with this chair. I assume he was upset regarding something in the game he was watching.

The registration clerk called 911, but the man left hospital property before officers could arrive. We tried to casually ask our patients about the man to see if he was there for them, but the closest we got was one patient seeming to acknowledge that he had a male visitor in the waiting area. The patient said, "If you're asking about him, that must mean he's done something wrong," and then refused to talk about the visitor further.

Since that night, the waiting area has been without a television. I don't think management has plans to replace it because they don't have to deal with the consequences of having bored, nervous, or angry patients and/or visitors in the waiting area without something to keep them occupied. We've seen a significant increase in fights in our waiting area since the television was broken, so I hope they get it fixed soon.

I am still in complete shock that someone would destroy a television over a football game!

Don't Mind if I Do

My patient 'kinda figured' she was pregnant because she hadn't had a menstrual cycle in 'a while.' She'd also been experiencing morning sickness, food aversions, breast tenderness, and mild cramping.

Her preg-test was positive, and we calculated that the patient was roughly nine weeks along. We used a doppler to detect fetal heartbeat.

As we were wrapping up in the room, the patient picked up the doppler and said, "Hey, this is cool. I need something like this."

She then put it in her backpack.

Our doctor sarcastically said, "Hey, I think someone left a cart unattended. Wanna go take all that stuff, too?"

The patient's eyes lit up.

Our doctor then told the patient to put the doppler back on the counter and (basically) get the hell out of our ER if she was going to come in and steal right in front of us.

I've only been employed here a year or so, so I don't have many shocking stories to submit. Our doctor said he's been with the hospital for more than a decade and that was the first time he's witnessed a patient doing something like that.

-J.A.
Arkansas

Back in the late-80s, early-90s, I had to make an arrest for a man doing something that went down as local history.

We'd recently experienced town-wide flooding, so most of our streets were impassable and officially closed off.

That didn't stop John from trying to get to the bar.

He 'borrowed' his neighbor's jet ski (by knocking a window out of a locked garage) and was found skiing down a flooded side street. He was already heavily intoxicated.

He was arrested following a complaint that he'd crashed into a utility pole.

-P.L.

Location withheld at request

Oh, Yeah!

Officers brought us an ETOH bar-fight patient who seemed antsy and paranoid. I made a reference to his behavior, but he assured me he was just nervous about being drunk and in the hospital.

It took all I had not to tell the patient, "Well, as soon as you're discharged you can be nervous about being drunk and in jail."

I had to leave the room and told the patient to sit tight, that I'd be back in a few minutes. The officers who'd brought the patient in were over at our station, grabbing snacks someone had brought in for my coworker's birthday. I had no reason to believe the patient was going anywhere. As I was leaving, I closed the door to the room, and I went about my business.

(At this point, I'm going to add that our ER was under construction, so some of our rooms were constructed of modular walls. These were sections of—I think—hard plastic framed by steel or some kind of metal. They were set up to look like rooms, but you couldn't see through the walls because they were made of solid material. The areas appeared sturdy, as the frames were bolted to the floor, and each treatment area had a door.)

I answered a call light or three, and I decided to grab a few chips before going back to the patient's room. As I was cramming Ruffles in my mouth and joking with the officers, we heard a crash.

Everyone in the ER looked over to see the ETOH patient lying on the floor. He'd come crashing through one of the panels like the Kool-Aid man!

The patient tried to run, but our exit was blocked off for construction. (We were re-routing our traffic to another exit on the opposite side of the room.) The confusion gave officers enough time to catch the patient. We had to give him a once-over, but he only had a few scratches.

When one of the officers asked the patient why he ran, he admitted that he had heroin on him, and he knew he would be in more trouble once he was taken to jail for processing and the officers found the drugs.

The officer asked, "So why didn't you just use the door, dipshit?"

The patient shrugged and said, "How was I supposed to know if it had an alarm or something?"

Our department head was pissed when she found out someone had destroyed part of the wall. She's the same person who shooed me out of her office for complaining about being assaulted by a patient during a shift, so the next time I saw her, I brought up the wall and said with a shrug, "Guess that's just part of the job, huh?"

-H.O.
California

Out of the Mouths of Babes

I answered a 911 call and a young child was on the line. I don't think he could've been older than three or four.

I asked, "Where's your mommy and daddy?"

He said, "Daddy, um, is at work."

I asked, "Okay, where's your mommy?"

He replied, "In the bathroom."

"Is she hurt?" I asked.

"No," he said. "She's pooping!"

I heard a voice in the background shout, "John, who are you talking to? You'd better not be playing with my phone again."

"Can you take the phone to your mommy?" I asked.

When the boy entered the bathroom and was handing off the phone, he shouted, "Ugh, it stinks in here!"

Poor woman confirmed she was using the restroom and didn't know her son had dialed 911. She seemed embarrassed by the situation, but then again, I think I would be as well. She promised it wouldn't happen again.

-K.E.
Kansas

The most infuriating case I've ever seen in my ED was a husband who'd brought his wife in one night. He suspected his wife was lying about how 'all women' have unwanted facial hair, and he wanted an 'expert opinion.'

This man pulled me aside and tried to slip me $20 to basically tell his wife that she had a one-of-a-kind problem and that other women don't have to wax or pluck hairs from their upper lips and/or chin. He told me he wanted her to feel bad because she did not look like a model on TV. He hoped this would convince her to 'change herself.'

I told the husband to get out of my ED, privately asked the wife (who appeared to be in great shape) if she was a domestic abuse victim. She said no, so then I assured her that her condition was normal and discharged her.

-R.R., M.D.
Arizona

Workplace Fun

Readers have sent in ways they've gotten a few laughs from coworkers. Here are a few:

It was my partner's first day to drive, so I squirted globs of KY Jelly all over the windshield and stuck a few leaves over the driver's side, so he'd be forced to turn on the wipers. He didn't understand why the 'gunk' on the windshield was smearing around, so we sat there for about six minutes with this guy in deep thought. I finally told him what the gunk was, and he just laughed and shook his head.

-K.M.
Kentucky

One of my coworkers and I had been in a prank war for a while. This is what made me surrender: He put packs of glitter in the vents on each side of the rig steering wheel, so when we started up the rig and the A/C blew, glitter exploded from the vents and covered me.

Nobody's been able to get in and out of that rig without finding glitter on them. It's been six months.

We were both written up for this, by the way, so I don't recommend doing it.

-J.H.
Minnesota

Our new tech said something about feeling left out, so we told her CS sent us the wrong batch of syringes and that we needed her to go down there and order more.

I can only imagine what the CS lady looked like when our tech went down there and told her that CS had sent us left-hand syringes and that we needed right-hand syringes.

-O.L.
Pennsylvania

I had been on vacation for two weeks. When I came back, I was called upstairs to float.

I got in the elevator and couldn't get the doors to close.

"Oh," my coworker said, "the buttons are all messed up. You have to hit them really hard. Maintenance knows, and they're gonna send someone to fix it this week."

I slapped the button, but the door wouldn't close.

"Gotta hit it harder," she said.

I smacked the button again, but the door still didn't close.

"No," my coworker said. "You really have to put your weight into it. Hit it hard."

I hit the button as hard as I could and screamed in frustration, "Why won't this thing close?"

My coworker started laughing and pulled out a sign she'd taken off the doors.

She said, "Because it's broken. We've had to use the stairs all week."

-D.W.
South Dakota

My 4-year-old grandson somehow put a ringtone (kittens crying) on my phone without my knowledge, and when I discovered he'd done it, my coworkers and I decided to have some fun.

We put my phone in the cabinet in our supply room and told the doctor, "We think there are kittens in the supply area, but we can't find them."

When he went in there, we kept calling my phone.

He was in there for 15 minutes before he found the phone and realized there were no kittens.

-H.E.
Montana

Our new guy was nervous, so we decided to break the ice and give him a proper welcome to the unit. It was flu season, so we told him that Lab had requested a vial of air from every floor in the hospital. We lied and said they were going to use some new machine to see if there were any signs of influenza in the air.

He was walking down the hall with a vial and cap like he was trying to catch butterflies for a good three minutes before we said that should suffice.

He laughed when he realized we were making crap up, but he got us back good by putting Vaseline on our phones.

-M.G.
Ohio

One of the guys said he'd switch shifts with me, but then he had to back out. There were no hard feelings because we've worked together for 12 years and are practically best friends.

I wanted to give him crap, though, so while he was in the bathroom, I took the straw out of his can of diet soda, cut the corner off a pack of soy sauce, taped the straw to it, stuffed the packet down into the can, and then I just sat at my desk and waited for him to come back.

He asked me why I was staring, but I just shrugged and said, "Guess I'm just day dreaming about the three-day weekend I can't have."

He laughed, took a huge sip from his straw, and spit soy sauce all over.

-J.W.
North Carolina

We noticed right away that our rookie was a kiss-ass, so we convinced him that our supervisor liked pickle and onion sandwiches.

This kid brought and ate pickle and onion sandwiches at lunch for four days and kept trying to find a way to bring up the sandwiches in conversations with our supervisor.

We finally told him we were just screwing around, but it was the funniest four days of my life.

-S.H.
Delaware

At the time, we only had one female employed at our station. She was pregnant and her doctor put her on light duty, so she went on desk and dispatch for a while. We gave her a bunch of crap about it, and she joked back.

Well one day, while we were waiting around for another call, she radioed me and said, "My water broke."

We're trained for this, and I think a few of us had even delivered before, but we were freaking out.

I ran in the room, only to find a bottle of water spilled on the floor.

We all laughed about it, but I was panicking before I realized she was joking.

-P.S.
Alabama

I was training for a marathon, and I noticed a girl from Peds had been losing weight steadily. I'd seen her mixing water in a shaker filled with orange powder, so one day I asked her what the powder was. She told me it was the cheese packet that comes in a box of macaroni.

I asked, "How does that even work?"

She shrugged and said she swore by it.

My dumb ass went to the grocery store before my shift, bought a box of macaroni, dumped the cheese packet in my own tumbler, and went to work. At lunch, I saw the girl from Peds filling up her shaker, so I filled up mine. We sat down at the same table in the lounge and took a swig from our cups at the same time.

I spit mine out; she did not.

I gagged and said, "Ugh, I don't know how you drink this stuff!"

She looked at me like I was nuts, started laughing, and said, "Jane, I was just kidding! This is a weight loss shake."

-L.T.
Louisiana

Author's Note: As I'm sure you're all aware, I do not condone hazing in the workplace, and I have no reason to believe these submissions were anything more than harmless pranks. If you plan to play pranks on your coworkers, you may want to check your facility's employee handbook first. Also, it's never a good idea to steal or 'borrow' equipment from your workplace, as this could be grounds for termination. Prank at your own risk.

The Story That Keeps on Giving

I remember quite well that it was rush hour when the man I'm going to tell you about came to the registration window. There had been a pileup on the freeway, and we were the nearest hospital, so I remember we were especially busy that day.

The man who'd walked in was wearing a torn, stained t-shirt and teeny tiny Daisy Duke shorts. He probably had the hairiest legs I've ever seen, and I'm almost positive that part of his penis was hanging out of one of the legs of the shorts. He was wearing a pair of mud-covered boots that came up to his knees.

I remember thinking, "Huh," and giggling a bit, but I didn't give it more thought. He'd noticed my reaction, though, I guess, so the first thing he said to me was, "These are my girlfriend's shorts."

I giggled again and said, "Okay. How can I help you?"

He growled, "Are you freaking kidding me?"

I then noticed the man only had one eyebrow.

I wasn't putting two and two together yet, so the man grew angrier. He waved a piece of duct tape at my window. His missing eyebrow appeared to be on the piece of tape.

He asked, "Can a doctor put this back on?"

I hesitated and then laughed because I thought he was joking. His stone expression made me straighten up.

"Sir," I said, "I don't think anyone here can replace your eyebrow."

He cussed a little, but then he turned around and stormed out without causing a scene. I could see his butt cheeks as he stomped out.

I'd say it was about a half hour later that we had a walk-in enter the lobby and approach the window. I think my coworkers and I all gasped, "Oh my God," simultaneously.

This man had a steak knife protruding from his side. His shirt was covered in blood. His face was bloody. One of my coworkers alerted Triage, so the man was whisked away to the magical world of emergency services.

Two officers arrived shortly after the patient was taken for treatment. We buzzed them back. A nurse called me from the back and told me to remain alert to the possibility that an armed man could enter ES. The man would be easy to spot because he would have a missing eyebrow. I passed this news to my coworkers and continued registering patients.

The nurse was correct in warning me to look out for the man in Daisy Dukes. However, he didn't come armed—he came in handcuffs. He was no longer wearing Daisy Dukes, but instead he was wearing crisp, brand-new jeans. I could tell they were brand-new because they still had the price sticker on the leg and the plastic security device on the waist.

Officers brought him to the window, and the man said, "I'm back."

"I see that," I said.

"Got busted for shoplifting," he casually told me, as if we were best friends catching up on the happenings of our lives.

"I see that, too," I said.

I asked, "Does this have something to do with your eyebrow?"

He grunted and muttered, "Yeah. Gonna kill the son of a bitch if I get my hands on him again."

I laughed nervously and said, "Man, you shouldn't say stuff like that when you're standing between two cops."

Anyway, I got the guy registered, and we gave the officers the first available open room. We try to stay on law enforcement's good side because we never know when we're going to need them. That's just one of the reasons.

I don't even think it was 15 minutes before our fire alarm was sounding and I saw one of our security guards running down the hall toward ES like he was trying to catch the last bus to Albuquerque. It looked like he was slipping on ice or something. I don't know if it was because the floor was still damp from where housekeeping had mopped, or if the guy's boots didn't have enough traction, but man, we thought he was gonna wipe out. It was crazy.

Someone from the back called us and told us *not* to evacuate, that the fire alarm was a false one.

Okay, but try telling that to a bunch of to-be-seen patients and visitors who thrive on total chaos.

There was a woman who was pacing the lobby, right in front of our window, frantically asking everyone walking out, "Hey, if you're leaving, can I have your place in line?"

Most people were ignoring her or saying no.

Once we calmed all these people down (we only had two or three LBTs), I went to the back to drop off someone's Chinese delivery and find out what the hell happened.

Security and police officers surrounded two rooms' doors. I could see the eyebrow guy in one room, cuffed to the bed rail. I saw a doctor examining stab guy's face. The stab guy's hands were stained with ink, so it was clear he'd pulled the fire alarm. Everyone was still in chaos mode, so it was hard to make heads or tails of anything.

I went back to my work area emptyhanded. My coworkers were so disappointed that I couldn't give them the scoop.

Probably about an hour-and-a-half into this cluster-f*ck, a woman came barging through the lobby, literally pushing people out of the way. She was dragging a duffle bag and was carrying a cardboard box. Her hair was a mess. Like, I don't even know how to describe it. Maybe she tried to dye her hair to look like a rainbow, but all the colors were splotchy. Her looked like a bokeh photo of Christmas lights on a tree. She was as thin as a twig. Someone could have farted as they were standing next to her and she probably would have blown away.

"Where's John?" she screamed at my coworker. She screamed threats at my coworker and started insulting my coworker's appearance and the like.

My coworker wasn't having any of this woman's sass, so she said sternly, "First of all, you need to check yourself. If you want any help at all, you'd better step back and wait your turn."

Well, that was like adding fuel to the fire. And BOOM!

The lady stepped back and dumped the contents of the box on the lobby floor. She was screaming, "You tell that mother-effer that I'm done with him. You hear me? I'm done! Don't be calling me. Better not show up at *my* house again, or I'll cut his nuts off. I'm done!"

She tried to throw the duffle bag, but I guess it was heavy or caught her shoulder just the right way, because everyone in the lobby heard a deafening popping sound, and then the lady started screaming her head off.

Triage stuck her head out from her room and then came out and examined the lady quickly, as in basically looked at the lady's shoulder for five seconds and said she probably dislocated her shoulder. She told the lady to register as a patient and then go to the waiting room and wait to be seen.

The lady flipped out even more and said, "Can't you see I'm hurt?"

Triage waved her arms around and said, "Can't you see that you're not the only patient in the emergency room today?"

The lady raised her good arm and acted like she was going to hit the Triage nurse, but the nurse didn't even flinch. She said to something like, "If you hit me, you'd better be prepared for me to hit you back."

I was 10 steps ahead of the situation and had already paged security. They sent one of the guards from the back part of ES and he stepped between the women to deescalate the situation. My coworker registered the lady at the desk, while the security guard started picking up the stuff on the floor.

As soon as my coworker registered the lady, we each instructed her to go to the waiting room. She finally turned to leave, but she saw that someone had picked up an item off the floor and was walking out with it. I'm not even sure what the item was. I thought it looked like one of those wax animals you get from those machines at the zoo, but I'm not sure.

The lady screamed at the man to put the item back, so he just grunted and tossed the item to the floor. Well, it hit the woman's foot, so she saw this as an attack on her, and she went rushing at him with her good arm extended like she was going to clothesline him if she could get him to turn just a little bit more to his side.

Our security guard grabbed her and told her to go sit down. She yelled at him, but she finally listened.

I don't know if I should say that I wish you could've heard all the screaming that went on when they finally called her back, or if you should be glad that you didn't have to hear any of it. I don't even know how to describe it. The lady was screaming like a wet cat at first, but then she sounded like she was possessed. Then we heard her crying and screaming. It was crazy.

Officers walked out with the first guy, Daisy Dukes. More officers walked in for the woman. A little bit later, we heard her scream, "What do you mean I'm pregnant?" Then, a little after that, we received a call that said stab guy was going to be admitted, so someone needed to come back and have him sign paperwork and all that.

I was curious to know the story, but I wasn't curious enough that I wanted to go to the guy's room, so my coworkers and I drew pencils from a cup that we kept on our desk specifically for moments like that. One of my coworkers drew the short pencil, so she had to go.

As she was coming back up to our workstation, after she'd spoken with stab guy, we heard the one lady scream like *she'd* been stabbed.

My other coworker kept her eyes on her paperwork and said, "They popped her shoulder back."

I nodded.

The coworker who'd gone to have paperwork signed told us the 'official, from the horse's mouth' (and in my opinion, totally bogus) story. I guess eyebrow guy and shoulder lady were sleeping together. Stab guy came home to find his girlfriend in bed with another man. He put duct tape over the guy's face and ripped off his eyebrow. Eyebrow guy woke up and the two started fighting, but then stab guy got distracted by shoulder lady. Eyebrow guy couldn't find his pants, so he put on shoulder lady's shorts and threw on some boots he'd found by the door. Stab guy was busy fighting with shoulder lady.

Eyebrow guy came to the ES and then sought out stab guy when he found out nobody could put his eyebrow back on his face. He beat and stabbed stab guy. From there—and I don't know the story, but I know enough of it—eyebrow guy apparently shoplifted from a store and was somehow apprehended shortly after. Stab guy told shoulder lady to move out of their rental home, and then he came to the ES. Shoulder lady was mad at stab guy, so she dumped his stuff in our lobby as a way to say she wasn't going to be the one to move out.

This is what I know happened for sure: In the back, when the two men saw each other, eyebrow guy went after stab guy, and stab guy pulled the fire alarm (accidentally, according to a nurse I talked to) before officers had a chance to step in.

Shoulder lady was taken to jail after she was seen, but I really don't know why. Stab guy had been discharged by the time I got to work the next day. No idea what happened to eyebrow guy.

I still don't believe anything the guy said about the time prior to the time he got to the hospital. I honestly think all three of these people were fighting about drugs or something, but I have no proof to base my opinion on. If it really went down the way stab guy said it did, then I have additional questions. First of all, I still want to know who walks in on their significant other asleep in bed with another lover and thinks, 'Hmm, I'll just rip his eyebrow off with duct tape.' I also want to know why eyebrow guy's first move was to get dressed and come to the hospital. Kinda want to know what was going through the lady's mind to think that stab guy should be the one to move out, but maybe there was more to that. I also want to know why shoulder lady was arrested.

All I know for sure is that 1.) One guy was dressed in hoochie shorts and was missing an eyebrow. 2.) One guy had been stabbed. 3.) They guys fought in the back, and stab guy pulled the fire alarm. 4.) The woman dumped a box of personal effects on the lobby floor and hurt herself. 5.) Two out of the three people went to jail.

Like I said, I think drugs were involved. Nobody ever mentioned drugs, but I honestly wouldn't be surprised if drugs had been involved.

My coworkers and I tried telling the other shifts about what happened, but half our coworkers weren't interested because our department makes everything into a competition of who has a harder job. The other half thought we were lying because every time we'd get to the next part, it'd be crazier than the part before.

To be fair, I completely understand why my coworkers would think we were lying. There's still so much of that story that sounds like total bull. If my coworkers had been the ones to tell me the story, I'm not sure I would have believed them. So many unanswered questions!

When that went down, I think I'd been in ES for about a year. I've been here a while now, but that was the most outrageous thing I've seen yet. I've seen a lot of crazy things, like a guy who'd come in because he thought he got herpes from his dog licking his face, and then a woman brought in by EMS because she took a bunch of drugs and beat the crap out of her bathroom mirror because she thought her reflection was her evil doppelganger trying to take over her life and trap her in the mirror.

-C.H.
California

We had a high guy walk in one night. He stood at the registration counter and kept trying to order food.

I think three different people told him about 800 times that he was in the emergency room, but he was really messed up and kept telling us to 'stop playing' because he just wanted to order his food and go back home.

The Unit Clerk from the back finally brought up a prepackaged sandwich and a carton of juice.

The guy put a bag of change on the counter and left.

Weirdest night ever.

-J.R.
Louisiana

The Calling

I love hearing from readers why they followed the healthcare/first responder path. Just when you think you know what type of answer you'll receive, one can jump out and surprise you. Here are the shortened versions of why some healthcare professionals and first responders chose this life:

When I was in first or second grade, we took a field trip to the hospital. PT had a wax bath for RA patients, and they let some of us dip our fingers in the wax. I thought becoming a nurse meant you got to stick your hands in wax all day.

-E.G.
Iowa

From a young age, I was fascinated with lights and sirens. Firetrucks were my favorite part of our local parades.

I'm proud to say that I've been with our station for 23 years.

The best part of my job, besides helping people, is getting to play with the lights and sirens.

-J.F.

New York

My dad worked as a janitor at our small-town hospital. He worked the overnight shift, so I'd go to school during the day, and then I'd go over to my aunt's house for a while. My dad would come get me and spend a few hours with me, and then he'd take me back to my aunt's. When it was time for her to go to work, she'd bring me to the hospital, and my dad let me sleep in one of the empty waiting rooms until it was time for us to go home, where he'd get me ready for school.

Sometimes, on the weekends, he'd give me quarters to get snacks from the vending machines, and then he'd let me sit in one of the waiting rooms and watch TV.

I didn't realize until I was older that my single dad risked his job by doing that. I also didn't realize he had to do that all those years because he couldn't afford a babysitter.

I kind of considered the hospital my second home, and that's why I went on to be a Med/Surg tech.

-M.T.
Location held at request

Money.

-K.E.
Hawaii

I spent a lot of time at my grandma's house when I was growing up. She was addicted to General Hospital. That show had me thinking that I could grow up and have the same kind of drama-filled life as the characters.

I have drama now, but not the 'Whisk me away to the breakroom for passionate kisses' kind. It's more like the, 'Stephanie, stop stealing my f*cking pens' kind.

-O.C.
Illinois

I thought wearing scrubs sounded better than wearing a business suit. I don't think people who wear business suits go home smelling like puke or C. diff.

-B.E.
Georgia

My mother's alcoholic ex broke into our house one night, and he started beating her. I thought she was going to die. I hid in the bathroom linen closet and used the cordless phone to call 911.

The dispatcher asked how old I was. I told her I was seven. She told me she had a daughter my age, and she started asking me questions about my favorite animals and my favorite color. She really helped me stay focused and when I'd get upset, she'd start talking to me about something else just to keep me calm. She gave the police officers a secret password to tell me, just so I'd know it was safe to come out of hiding.

Growing up, I knew I wanted to do that for other people. I hope I make other people feel as safe as that dispatcher made me feel.

-U.K.
Ohio

My mom said I have always been concerned about others' wellbeing. She said that even when I was a baby and my cousin bumped his head, that I kissed the bump to make it better, much like my mother did with my ouchies.

As a child, I started a pretend clinic for my toys. I lined all my dolls and teddy bears in the waiting room (my closet), and then I would call them individually and perform surgeries on my bedroom floor. They went to 'recovery' (my bed) soon after their surgeries.

I became CPR certified in fourth grade, after our health teacher taught a lesson on first aid. I fished my brother out of the pool a year later and saved his life with the CPR I'd learned in health class.

In high school, I attended dual-credit classes, which allowed me to graduate with a degree in nursing. I went on to university and now have the N.P. initials following my name.

I can't remember a time in my life when I did not feel a strong connection with the medical world. I honestly feel that I was born to do this. My parents joke that I was probably a nurse in another life, and I can't disagree. This is all I've ever wanted. I live and breathe for helping others.

-J.E.-P., N.P.

When I was about four or five, I somehow got my head stuck in the porch railing. My mom called 911. Two medics spent about 30 minutes freeing me.

I grew up and realized how that would be a wild way to spend the day, so I became certified.

None of my calls are like that, unfortunately.

-G.H.
Rhode Island

I love older people, but I'm not cut out for nursing. I work in the kitchen at an SNF and love being able to see our residents. You can really tell when someone's lonely because they look forward to routines like meals, and they always have a smile when they see you. I really picked the best place to work, too, because everyone here respects one another as equals, so we're all one big family here to give the residents a great place to stay.

-A.G.
Maine

We used to go see my Pop-Pop at the nursing home. (Our house wasn't big enough for him to live with us, and it wasn't up to code for the type of care he'd need, nor could my mom and dad afford a live-in nurse.) We'd sit with Pop-Pop for hours when we'd visit. This old man across the hall would always sit in his rocking chair and just stair into Pop-Pop's room. I was young, and it made me feel uncomfortable.

One day, we arrived in Pop-Pop's room, and the nursing staff had moved the old man's rocking chair into my grandfather's room.

Pop-Pop explained that his neighbor never had visitors and was lonely. His neighbor saw how much we'd laugh and talk, so he asked Pop-Pop if he could come over during some of our visits, just so he could feel included.

We 'adopted' him as our second Pop-Pop and brought him Christmas gifts and snacks and we all played games together.

I started volunteering at the hospital when I was 16. I'm in my 40s now, and I still volunteer religiously because I never want anyone to feel alone. I read to patients, sing with them, and I look at countless pictures of relatives who never come to visit. One of my patients even taught me how to knit booties for my grandson. I wouldn't trade volunteering for the world.

-C.A.
Maine

911 call to a sorority house.

A female got her tongue stuck in the opening of a wine bottle.

After we got the young woman free, she gazed up at me with her glossy eyes, without a care in the world that she had a merlot ring around her mouth, and she vomited on the carpet.

-H.H.
Florida

I thought I was having a bad day until I removed my homeless patient's boots. When I peeled off his socks, most of his skin came off. What's worse is that one of his toes fell off in my hand.

-A.K.
New York

Inked

Years ago, I responded to an altercation at a park. When I arrived, bystanders were restraining two male subjects.

When I asked the men to explain, one male said, "He was trying to steal my life!"

"Like, kill you?" I asked.

He shook his head and removed his shirt. When he turned around, I noticed a series of numbers tattooed across his back.

"Is that your social security number?" I asked.

"Yes!" he said. "And he," the man shouted, while pointing at the other male, "was writing it down while I was playing basketball. I had to put my shirt back on!"

"I was not," the second male argued. "I already told you I didn't. I even offered to show you my notebook."

The bystanders thought that because an officer was present that the situation was secure, but once the men started scrapping again, it was clear the situation was not under control. We managed to pull the men apart again.

"Did you write down his information?" I asked the second male.

"No!"

I asked, "Mind if I look through your notebook? Maybe ask you to empty your pockets to see if you wrote it down and put the paper in your pocket?"

This man agreed. His notebook was filled with sketches of people in motion. He explained he was in art school, and he was studying various sports and dancing techniques to piece together his final project.

"It doesn't look like he wrote it down," I said to the first male.

"And you better not ever," the first man shouted to the second. "That's private information!"

"Sir," I said, "it's not so private if you have it tattooed on your back and are playing basketball with your shirt off."

"Are you gonna arrest him?" the first male asked.

I shook my head and said I figured we could chalk it up to a simple disagreement, as long as both parties agreed.

The first man wasn't hearing it, so I said, "Well, all these witnesses said you threw the first punch. So, it sounds like you would be the one going to jail. As far as I can tell, this gentleman was within his rights to defend himself."

Say something like that and everyone becomes willing to let bygones be bygones.

The second male asked if he could leave, so I told him that was fine.

"What were those other things tattooed on you?" I asked the first male.

He turned around and let me take a look. He had his blood type, date of birth, and three different addresses tattooed on his back in smaller print. It appeared that when he moved from one address to the next, he would have his tattoo artist tattoo a line through the previous address.

"Why would you do that?" I asked.

He shrugged and said, "In case I die, and they find me in the alley or something."

I couldn't help but to ask him, "Do you participate in many dangerous activities that you think you need a tattoo like that to identify you?"

He shrugged and said, "Well, I do blow."

I laughed, rubbed my eyes, and muttered, "Oh my God."

I told the man to stay out of trouble and to keep his shirt on if he didn't want someone trying to 'steal his life.'

I never heard anyone else talking about him, and I don't recall ever seeing a headline of the body of a man with his SSN tattooed across his back being discovered in an alley, so maybe he's still out there somewhere.

-J.I.
Illinois

Counting only *my* patients, last year there were 22 cases of new parents in our ED for a complaint that their child/children were caught eating cat/dog/ferret food.

A parent with five children overheard my new parents leaving with their twins and told them with a laugh, "Once you get to kid number three, you'll see them eating out of the dog bowl and count that as dinner."

-R.G.
New York

Act of Kindness

We once had a woman who donated a bunch of blankets, hats, and stuffed animals to our floor, a pediatric oncology wing. She crocheted the blankets, folded them in squares, and then tied them up with ribbons. She added a card with each blanket. I think the cards had her name and a prayer typed on them.

Since our patients receive donations like this often, we didn't think too much of it. We were grateful, don't get me wrong. I should rephrase and explain that we did not believe this would be problematic. Geeze Louise were we ever wrong.

About a month after the woman donated the blankets, she came back. We thought she wanted to donate more items, but instead she asked if it would be okay to visit some of the patients who'd received the donations. Most parents agreed to this, as we believed the woman just wanted to see how much joy her donations brought to the children.

When she entered the first room, none of our staff was present. We heard one of the mothers saying to the patient's grandma, "Well, that was just rude." Later on, it was revealed that the woman who'd donated interrogated the child because the child did not have one of her blankets, hats, or stuffed animals with him.

I think it was on the third room that the woman entered that we realized it was time for her to go. We could hear her shouting from the end of the hall.

When my coworker and I entered the room, our patient—a female between the ages of 4 and 8—was sobbing. The child's father was standing between the bed and the woman. The child was clinging to one of the blankets that had been donated. The woman who'd donated the blanket was trying to rip the blanket from the child's arms.

We asked what was going on, and that's when the woman got in my coworker's face and began berating us for allowing the blankets to be 'ruined.' She said the blankets were never meant to be used or washed, and that the items she'd donated were for publicity only. She wanted the parents to post pictures of the items online so her shop could get free publicity and that 'anyone with half a brain' could figure out that 'cancer kids get lots of attention.'

This woman was livid, absolutely livid, that *her* blankets had gone through the wash or had been snagged or were actually being used by our patients. She then hit my coworker.

While I had my head sticking out the patient's room, screaming hysterically for *anyone* to call security, the only thought it my mind was, 'Thank God she didn't see John's stuffed bear.' We gave John clearance to try to keep down fruit punch— the only food or drink the toddler would show the faintest interest in after his latest round of treatment— but that didn't end so well. John's teddy bear started out as white, but no amount of washing could get the red vomit out of it, so his mom threw it in the trash.

We couldn't wait around for security, so an orderly and a tech dragged the woman out of the patient's room. She still had a tuft of my coworker's hair in her hands as she was restrained in the hallway.

The incident was reported to administration immediately. It was also reported to law enforcement. The hospital banned the woman from the property, excluding healthcare visits.

I think it was about a week or so later that we heard she'd checked herself into the ER. We didn't even know she was on hospital property until staff caught her in the stairwell. I don't know with certainty that she was headed to our floor, but she *was* only three floors down, so I don't know.

Our kids were as good as we could expect. We allowed the children to keep the donated items (if the children wanted them and the parents allowed the children to keep them).

That incident left a sour taste in my mouth. Our patients already have difficult lives, and they're only children. People often underestimate the impact these types of donations can have on our patients' well-being.

This happened a long time ago, but I still sometimes want to track the woman down and scream in her face, "WTF is wrong with you?!"

-K.E.
Texas

Bad Bosses

We've all had 'em. Some of us probably have 'em now. Readers share reasons why their bosses are/were horrible.

We have two supervisors. Both made the Christmas party mandatory, but they refused to supply funds for the party. They offered us use of one of the conference rooms after hours, but otherwise, it was our 'responsibility' to furnish snacks, decorations, and entertainment.

They didn't give us a list of items we *couldn't* bring, so my coworkers and I spent $200 on alcohol and two of our boyfriends volunteered to be our DDs. We sat in the conference room, watched Lifetime movies, and got hammered.

Our supervisors didn't even show up to their own department 'party' because they're crappy people. It's probably for the best because none of us can stand them, anyway.

-B.T.

Indiana

My mother died some years ago. It was quite unexpected, as she was so young. She was involved in an MVA caused by a drunk driver.

When I rang my boss and explained I needed to take time off to make arrangements, he said, "That's fine. You have two days off coming up. That should be enough time."

I asked, "Huh?"

"Saturday and Sunday," he said, laughing. "Those are your days off. Take care of your business on your scheduled days, like everyone else has to do."

I had to file a formal complaint to get the time off, and from that time on, I had to file complaints through Human Resources to get *any* time off.

-S.L.
Ohio

My boss fired me for losing the keys to the supply closet, despite me telling him that I never even *had* the keys to the supply closet.

My former coworker texted me a few days later and said they found the keys under the work fridge.

I never even got an apology.

-R.L.
Tennessee

With literally two minutes (!) left of my shift at the station, my husband dropped my daughter off so he could go to work. This was a one-time occurrence.

I was fired on the spot because 'work is not a daycare.'

I decided to use this in my favor, so I went back to school for certification. My daycare business pays me triple what I was making at the station.

What's even more hilarious is that my former boss pays me to watch his children because every other daycare was filled up.

-A.M.
Idaho

After working in ER for 19 years, I wanted to try a different change of pace. I applied for a shoo-in department that was having difficulty keeping RNs, so I knew my transfer would be accepted immediately. It was not. Dismayed, I tried for two other departments. They also declined my transfer.

I noticed my schedule became wonky surrounding my transfer requests. At first, I didn't say anything because I appreciate all the overtime I can get. When my supervisor approached me and said something about, "I bet you're tired," I just shrugged it off and told her what I just told you. Two days later, I was cut on the schedule to the bare minimum requirement for hours. This went on for weeks.

The last straw was when I had spoken to our scheduler about scheduling one of my days off for my granddaughter's Christening. She approved it, but days later I noticed I was scheduled for that day. When I asked the scheduler she said, "I don't know. That's just what [ER supervisor] told me to change it to."

I decided to dig around a bit. I knew I hadn't been the only one in all my years with the ER who'd had trouble transferring. The difference was that most of my coworkers had either given up on their dreams of transferring, or they quit and went to different hospitals. I was determined to stay with our facility, but I wanted out of ER.

After speaking with the department supervisor about the shoo-in position, she let it slip that the ER supervisor had dragged my character through the mud. I was fuming, but I had no concrete evidence to support my claims, and I knew I couldn't take my claims to H.R. because the shoo-in's supervisor was unlikely to testify on what she'd accidentally told me.

The next time there was an opening on another floor, I kept my intentions to myself, spoke personally with the department head, and I submitted all my transfer requests via hard-copy paperwork, rather than using our electronic transfer request system. I was accepted.

The ER supervisor was pissed and tried to get me fired for 'going behind her back' to request a position in another department. H.R. concluded that I had done nothing wrong. A short time later, a group of people had come forward with evidence that the ER head had been tampering with requests, slandering employees to inquiring supervisors, and was basically doing everything she could to not only keep RNs in the ER, but also make them hate their lives if they attempted a transfer.

I am happy to tell you that I now work on a Psych unit and have not had an ounce of trouble from any of my coworkers or head supervisor. I wish I would have known that working in other departments could be this good. I spent 19 years in the ER thinking 'this is just how it is at this hospital,' when in reality, that's just how it was working in that department.

-T.M.
Ohio

(Author's Note: Unfortunately, I can tell you many stories like this, and I can bet most of our readers have similar stories.)

One of our volunteers had a disability. Our Director called him [R-word] to his face, and then turned to us, laughing and said, "It's not like he can understand what I'm saying, anyway."

Every last person who was present filed formal complaints. Our Director was walked out by security and was permanently trespassed from the premises.

-M.S.
Location withheld at request

Our office had a staff appreciation day. They provided two $3 boxes of juice barrel drinks. The email asked us to bring everything else. So, really, we just had an employee-funded potluck to remind us that we were 'so appreciated' that our bosses were too cheap to order us pizza or something.

-E.K.
Delaware

We had a mom bring in a mud-covered pre-teen one day. She said he was out with her 'bastard ex-husband,' who decided to take the child 'mudding' on ATVs.

Mom not only wanted the child checked out for physical injuries, but she also demanded that we utilize our decon shower and send her ex the bill, since (and I quote), "Mud can kill you."

I still shudder to think of what type of relationship (or lack thereof) the child is watching his parents have.

By the way, the kid was perfectly fine.

-A.C.-H.
Iowa

When Life Gives You Lemons

"Sir," I asked the man in the ED lobby, "is there any particular reason you're pushing around an orange tree in a wheelchair?"

"It's a *lemon* tree," he corrected. "And I had to bring it inside because if I left it in the bed of my truck, someone would steal it."

"Okay," I replied. "Why don't you have a seat, and we'll call you as soon as your name pops up."

The registration guy whispered to me, "That's the chest pain I called you about."

Registration babysat the 3 to 4-foot tree while we whisked its owner to a room.

-D.S.
California

Have a Seat

Picture it: 03:45. An eerily-quiet emergency room, dimly illuminated by soft white lights embedded in the walls, as not a single patient had graced us with their presence. Soft laughter erupted intermittently from the back, as nurses and doctors wrapped in warm blankets huddled around Jane's laptop to watch YouTube videos. Up front, on the exhausted registrar's laptop, an episode of Black Mirror played.

Suddenly, the phone rang. The registrar answered with a yawn, as she recognized the number as one from the back.

"Come to the back," the voice said. "We stole a box of cookies from Rehab, and we found some hot chocolate."

Never one to pass up cookies *or* hot chocolate, the registrar hurried to the back. If she'd learned anything in her two years of employment at a hospital, it was this: One can never dilly-dally when food is present, or it will be gone by the time you get there.

So, yours truly loaded up on cookies. The hot chocolate was the kind without marshmallows, so I improvised. I found a box of smores Goldfish in the cabinet and dropped some dehydrated marshmallows in my cup. I wasn't entirely sure how it'd taste, but I was willing to take my chances.

I bid farewell to the group of nurses and doctors, as I continued to my work station to continue my episode of Black Mirror.

With a mere three feet to go, the emergency alarm blared. I jumped so high I think my cookies touched the ceiling before they fell to the floor. I never had the opportunity to test my ingenious idea of Goldfish marshmallows in hot chocolate because I dropped the cup.

"Don't slip on that!" I warned to the three nurses sprinting in my direction. "Go around! Go around!"

As I scavenged for paper towels to place over my mess, the nurses rushed outside. When the doors slid open, I heard, "We can't carry him anymore."

That bit of dialogue told me ignore the mess on the floor and get to my station to prepare for registration. It could be serious. Had it been raining? Perhaps the roads were slippery, which caused an MVA. Perhaps an elderly man fell down the stairs. The possibilities were endless.

"Why would you even do this?" one of the nurses shouted. "Who does something like this?"

"I know!" a male shouted back. "I thought it would be funny!"

Oh, now I *had* to stand up and look.

What the hell is wrong with people? Really, what—is—wrong—with—people?

This guy was old enough to know better. He probably had a wife or a husband or a significant other who was probably going to knock him upside the head for being in the emergency room for this.

Imagine a plastic patio chair, the rigid kind that does not fold. This one was white. Come to think of it, I'm not sure I've seen them in any other color. Green, maybe, not sure.

The patient was seated in the chair, but not properly. The chair was turned backwards, and the man had placed his legs through the arm holes. His legs were stuck. He was kind of on the big side.

He tried to lift his body up and walk, but he looked like a drunk crab. I think he fell over twice before one of the nurses sternly said, "Stop doing that!"

The patient was registered, and the nurses had to borrow a saw from Maintenance. Due to hospital policy, only Maintenance employees are permitted to operate the power tools that belong to the department, so nurses held the man's skin out of the way so Maintenance could cut the patient free.

This patient stated he was not under the influence of drugs and/or alcohol. He asked if he could take the chair with him, and of course we all obliged because it was not our chair to begin. Quite honestly, we have no need for another broken chair in our department, as we already have three. (I hope someone from our hospital reads this because I demand new chairs.)

Unfortunately, this patient opened the floodgates. More patients rushed in soon after he was registered. I think my hot chocolate and cookies remained on the floor for an hour. A housekeeper was walking through to begin her shift, saw the 'Wet Floor' sign I'd placed atop the (now) soggy paper towels and crushed Keebler's, and told me she would be back right away. God bless her because I'm not sure where I would have found the time to clean up after myself.

That was the first and only time during my employment with this hospital that we went almost four hours without seeing a patient. I miss it.

-L.H.
Kentucky

Pure Panic

We had a surprise visit from JCAHO. Technically, it wasn't a surprise to *everyone*. Higher ups knew they were coming, but they were evil and wanted to 'keep us on our toes,' so they neglected to pass along the information until the team entered the lobby. I guess registration speed-dialed someone back here.

I was the last one to hear about this because I was tending to a patient, but as soon as I caught wind, I grabbed my bottles of soda and water, and three bags of snacks and *bolted* toward the break room.

My clog slipped off, which started it all. I fell, landed on my soda bottle…which shot the lid off the bottle. The lid hit the wall right around the time my forehead bounced off the floor. My bottle of water rolled into a patient's room and was under the bed. I recovered two of my snack bags, but I couldn't find my bag of carrots. (They were later found behind a trash can.)

I thought my wrist was broken, so I had to register as a patient. What's worse is that I couldn't even lie my way out of the situation.

My wrist, thankfully, was not broken.

-C.U.
Location withheld at request

K.P. and J.H. from California sounding off:

We've had more than one patient and/or patient family wanting to name the new baby 'Chlamydia.' Most have commented to us that the name is 'pretty' or 'sounds exotic.'

If this means something in another language, we're not sure. The instances we recall involve patients and/or families of varied ethnicities, so I think these have been cases where the families either don't know what this word means, or they are so overjoyed with the new baby that their brains aren't putting two and two together.

All the times, we've just kind of nodded and smiled, but we do politely inform the families of the meaning we know for the word. None of *our* patients have gone through with this name, but we Googled it and found it's happened before, at least allegedly.

Ruh-Roh

My last patient of my ER employment was checking him/herself in. Our conversation went something like this:

Me: How can I help you?

Patient: There's gotta be something wrong with me.

Me: Uh, okay.

Patient: How many people can you name from Scooby-Doo?

Me: Uh…

Patient: Seriously. This is a serious question. I think I'm going insane.

Me: Uh… Would you like to speak with a doctor?

Patient: I think so, but I need you to answer my question first. How many people can you name from Scooby-Doo? And, like, I mean the main group. Not secondary characters or anything.

Me: Uh…

Patient: Tell me you remember that show.

Me: Yeah, I do, but… Are you kidding me?

Patient: This isn't a joke. I think something's broken in my brain. Just tell me who you remember, and then I'll tell you who I remember.

Me: Uh, okay. So, um, Scooby and Shaggy. Fred and Daphne. And, uh, the library woman with the glasses.

Patient: Velma.

Me: Yeah, that was her name.

Patient: But you don't remember anyone else?

Me: Oh, that teeny tiny Scooby. His cousin or something.

Patient: No, Scrappy was a secondary character. And he was Scooby's nephew, not his cousin.

Me: Uh, okay. Yeah, I haven't watched that show in years.

Patient: But you don't remember anyone else?

Me: Uh… No? Should I?

Patient: Well, don't you think it's kind of weird that Scoob and Shaggy were partners, and then Fred and Daphne were partners?

Me: Uh…

Patient: Everyone I talk to says exactly what you said. They said they can't remember anyone else.

Me: Do you need to see a doctor?

Patient: Yeah, I think I do. I remember a different show.

Me: Other than Scooby-Doo?

Patient: No. That's what I'm telling you. My memories are the right ones. I thought so, anyway. But I started talking to someone about it, and they said I must've been confused. But I'm not confused. I know that I spent almost my entire childhood and teenage years and even watched it in college, and I remember that Velma had a partner.

Me: We'll get you registered.

Patient: But you're serious? You really don't remember there being another character? Like, he was in almost every single episode. You don't remember that?

Me: Uh, no. But, like I said, I haven't watched that show in years.

Patient: Maybe I fell asleep and woke up in a different timeline.

Me: Uh, possibly. Let's get you registered.

-I.L.
Washington

He Chose Poorly

I once had a patient give me a fake name at registration.

It *may* have worked if he'd not hesitated for at least a minute before giving me one of the most popular names in film history.

When I busted him, he said, "Holy crap, you've seen those movies?"

"Yeah," I said. "Me and about ten million other people."

He told me his name was Indiana Jones.

Idiot.

-S.B.
New Jersey

Measurably Unexpected

My son was grounded for hitting his brother, so he was banned from video games, television, his cell phone, and any other electronic devices. He'd taken it upon himself to make the punishment work in his favor, but I wasn't giving in so easily. His plan, I do believe, was to annoy me so much that I'd tell him to go watch television.

He found my husband's tape measure and was going around the house measuring everything, including the width and height of the dog dishes, our appliances, the cat, and the kitchen table. He then began rolling out the measuring tape to see how far he could get it to expand without folding in on itself. It was getting on my nerves because every few seconds I'd hear the metal crinkling, the tape sliding back, and the bracket on the end slapping against the tape's hard case.

Right as I was about to holler at him, the tape folded in on itself, slid back, and my son dropped the tape measure on the floor. I noticed the blood before I realized he was screaming.

I called for my husband while I was wrapping a kitchen towel over my son's hand. My husband had to drive because I was in a state of panic.

My son had to get 11 sutures to close a wound that stretched from the tip of his pinky to his wrist.

Never in a million years did I think this could happen. I've never even *heard* of anyone else being injured from a tape measure, but the nursing staff assured me that this is a common injury in their department. Who knew?!

-D.C.
Georgia

Saving the World

My new partner and I went through a drive-thru for lunch. We parked and ate in the car.

I was putting my trash in the bag, when I saw my partner tearing up his fast food napkin and placing the strips in his mouth. I just watched, dumbfounded, as he ate an entire napkin.

"Man…" I asked. "Why'd you do that?!"

He looked at me like I was insane and said, "Uh, hello? They're biodegradable. That's what you're *supposed* to do with them."

At first, I thought he was messing with me, but he's eaten at least four napkins while we've worked together.

I'm not sure he understands what that word means, but I'm not gonna be the one to tell him. I'm just waiting for him to do it in front of someone else, just so I can see both of their reactions (if the other person asks about it).

-G.P.
Utah

Gallagher: Live in the ER

A few years ago, during our busiest day shift of the month, a heavily-pregnant woman and her partner came in to be seen for her complaint of 'itchy nose.' Half the people in our waiting room had complaints of vomiting and other flu-like symptoms, while the other half were bleeding and/or injured. I was internally screaming at this woman for wasting our time with such a stupid complaint. I sent her and her partner to the waiting room and told them it would be at least an hour before someone would call them back. They seemed agitated right off the bat. Whatever.

Well, about 15 minutes into their wait, the couple started arguing in the waiting room. I had to go in there and warn them to keep it down, or I'd be forced to call security. They talked some smack to me, but then they promised to keep quiet.

No sooner than I returned to my booth, the two were at it again. They were screaming at the top of their lungs. I called security.

As I was registering another patient, I saw the male grab the woman by her hair and pull her out of her chair. I started to call 911. At this point, I realized nobody in the waiting room had stepped in to help the woman. I could see at least one man recording the incident on his phone. I was disgusted.

I heard people screaming, and I saw the man with something in his hand. I couldn't quite tell what it was. I hung up on 911 and ran to the waiting room. I don't know what I planned to do because I am just over 5-feet tall, and I'm 110-pounds. The male was tall and muscular. I knew a few self defense moves, but all those moves were for scenarios where a guy would grab me from behind. I just knew that I had to do something because it was clear nobody else was going to do anything. I lost my best friend to domestic violence, and it's something that 'triggers' me. I sometimes have panic attacks if I even see domestic violence on television.

Right as I walked to the waiting room doorway, I saw the man draw back his arm. He was holding a hammer. I didn't even know where he'd gotten a hammer, but that didn't matter at the time.

I closed my eyes and screamed as the man hit the pregnant woman in the belly. A bunch of other people screamed too, but then I heard giggling.

When I dared to open my eyes, I noticed the man who'd been recording had his phone pointed at me, and then he panned around the room.

The 'pregnant' woman and her partner were laughing hysterically, and there was a busted watermelon all over the waiting room floor.

Security and the police arrived around the same time, and the two were arrested. I'm not sure what their charges were because I was too busy crying in the employee bathroom.

I guess the two had planned on performing this 'prank' in a treatment room, but when they were told it would be at least an hour before they'd be seen, they decided to do it right there in the waiting room. The guy recording was in on it.

I've seen burn patients, drug addicts, alcoholics who've chopped off limbs, and children who've suffered from life-threatening injuries or abuse. But this 'prank' has been the most terrifying thing I've seen while working at in healthcare.

-Initials and location withheld at request

Never Would Have Thought...

I want to contribute a story to your series in hope that it will prevent any person from becoming a patient for this reason.

Being a nightshift ES nurse with three children, three cats, and a husband, I seek to save time in any way imaginable. I meal prep on my days off, use grocery delivery apps, and for a long time, I used a hair removal cream to save time in the shower. I used this cream for years—at least five years—religiously. It worked like a charm.

Printed on the label is a warning for consumers. This warning recommends the consumer perform a skin patch test prior to applying the product for use on widespread areas. I performed this test when I began using the product. And, since I had no adverse reaction to the area which I had applied the cream, I continued using it without hesitation.

A few months ago, I used the product as part of my schedule. After the product has been applied, it is usual (at least in my case) to feel a slight tingling feeling. My legs also itch while the cream is applied. I noticed, however, a slight burning sensation. At first, I shrugged off the sensation, believing the temperature in the bathroom was too cold and the sensation was simply psychological. Seconds later, the burning sensation became unbearable. I rushed into the shower, scrubbed the cream off with a washrag, and was in total shock because the burning sensation had not subsided.

In addition to the burning sensation, I noticed my legs were red, as if I had bathed in scorching water. I had not. Upon leaving the shower and drying myself, I noticed my legs appeared swollen. I inspected myself in the mirror. I looked like a lobster, my skin was so red.

My first reaction was to pull out my old bottle from under the sink. I compared that label to the one on the new bottle. I even called the company and was on hold for a short amount of time, while the representative investigated any possible ingredient changes to the chemicals in the cream.

As time passed, the burning sensation worsened, and my legs felt heavy. I knew this was more than a simple chemical reaction, so I called my mother and asked her to drive me to my place of employment. I did not want to drag my husband and children along for the ride. Admittedly, I also did not want to listen to any of them gripe during our time spent at the ES, especially because it was my day off and they were tired, as this occurred later in the evening. I wanted peace and quiet for once.

The examination concluded that this appeared to be an allergic reaction to the cream itself. But how? I used the product as instructed. I had already done the patch test. I had used the product for years.

Our physician recommended that I try another patch test on my forearm, using cream from the old bottle. If I experienced a similar reaction, we could assume I was experiencing an allergic reaction. If I did not, we could assume the cream's ingredients had been altered.

Back at home, after a tiring ES visit, I conducted a skin test as recommended. My skin reacted in the same manner! Somehow, over the course of years, I had slowly developed an intolerance to the cream.

I have heard of this occurring in patients, usually when food is concerned. I have never seen a case as severe as mine, at least not in person.

I urge you and everyone else to please perform a patch test prior to applying these hair removal creams, lotions, and hair dyes—even if you've used them before. This may prevent you or others from experiencing results much worse than mine.

-I.G.
Wisconsin

Mistakes Were Made

Our ER is located in a bustling urban area. We see upwards of 100-150 patients per shift, and I'd say that's on an average day. On a busy day, the number can be close to 200.

This was a busy day. I had been called in early, and like you, I worked night shift. It threw off my internal balance to be awake and at work while the sun was still shining outside. I had gotten very little sleep, so I was exhausted. My supervisor told me if I came in early, I could leave at 02:00, so it was about 17:30 and I was counting down the hours as I sucked down coffee after coffee after coffee.

I went to the lobby and glanced at my paperwork. I looked at the registration clerks and asked angrily, "Is this some kind of joke?"

"What?" one of the young girls asked innocently.

"Never mind," I said, sighing loudly.

I called out, "Jesus?"

My brain was so beaten up that I wasn't pronouncing it like I have pronounced it so many times before. I was pronouncing it like you hear in church.

"Jesus?" I called louder. "Is there someone here named Jesus?"

Patients in the waiting room kind of snickered, and I felt like I was being set up. I stomped over to the registration area and confronted one of the clerks.

"Who did this?" I demanded.

"Did what?" the gentleman asked.

"Don't play stupid," I barked. "You picked the wrong nurse to play a joke on."

He said calmly, "I have no idea what you're talking about."

"Jesus!" I screamed. "You entered a patient's name as Jesus! When's the last time you've met someone named Jesus? What is wrong with you?"

"Hey," said another clerk, "I registered that patient."

"Are you stupid?" I asked. "What's next? Are you going to register Mickey Mouse next?"

The clerks all looked at me like I was an idiot, and rightfully so.

"It's *Jesús*," the female clerk said to me.

I felt so dumb! I have pronounced this name correctly a trillion times. I apologized profusely to the registration clerks, and then I began laughing and couldn't stop.

I had to go back to the waiting room and call out the name again, this time with its proper pronunciation.

I blamed the blunder on what it was: sleepiness.

I felt so bad for yelling at the registration crew that I ordered them pizza.

-K.B.
Nevada

Despicable

Several years ago, when I was a child, my grandmother lived with our family. She suffered from dementia and required around-the-clock care. Because my mother was a SAHM and housewife, she also cared for my grandmother. Grandma could move, but she required assistance, as she was prone to falls and often became confused. Once, my grandmother had gotten up in the middle of the night and had let our family's chihuahuas outside. Thankfully, my family had heard the commotion. Grandma, dressed in nothing more than a nightgown, said she was going to take the dogs to the dog park. We brought our dogs in from the blizzard outside and explained to Grandma that it was 02:00 in the morning and the weather was terrible.

I think I was 11 or 12 when my dad won a contest at work. He was awarded tickets for a Florida resort getaway. I think the tickets were good for three nights, and all travel and expenses were covered. It was a big deal in our house because we weren't living in poverty, but we weren't exactly high-class, either. We had steaks for dinner every few weeks, but we also used sandwich bread as hot dog buns. I had a bike that my mom had spotted in someone's trash. My dad painted it and said it looked new. While everyone else at school ate Lunchables with cookies and Capri Suns from their fancy Rugrats totes, I had a brown paper bag of PB & fluff sandwich, a baggy of off-brand BBQ chips, and paid for my milk with quarters my dad and I found on the ground by the vacuum cleaners at local car washes (we went around town almost every other day to do this).

My mom and dad looked at their budget, and they decided that since this was a once-in-a-lifetime opportunity for a family vacation, they would empty their savings to hire someone to stay with my Grandma. They contacted a small nursing service out of the newspaper and hired a help-at-home type of nurse. My mom was nervous at first, but the people on the phone were polite.

Mom and dad used most of their savings to pay the nursing service, and then they planned a few extra days to drive to Florida, rather than fly. The plan was to visit family along the way. Rather than a three or four-day trip, we were going to be gone seven days.

As you can imagine, this was a big deal. The trip was taking place in the middle of Autumn, and I had school. I thought I was such a hot shot. I walked around school thinking I was badass because I was getting about a weeks' worth of homework in advance (which I'd end up doing in the car or before bed each night). I was bragging to all my friends about all the cool things we were going to do. My friends and I were stupid, so a bunch of 10, 11, & 12-year old girls were sitting around talking about how I was going to find a 'hunk' like one of the Backstreet Boys when we were at the resort.

We drove through several states, visiting family along the way. We stopped at a few touristy places, but I think we were all ready for Florida. My mom had made it a point to give the nursing service phone numbers for every relative we'd planned to stop to see, as well as give the service the number for the resort. I know my mom called our house on the first night, for sure, and then maybe it was the second night too. The nurse assured my mom that 'everything was fine.' I do recall that on day three, my mom called late at night (once we reached another relative's house), but nobody answered. My dad told my mom that everyone was probably asleep.

On day four, my mom called throughout the day. No answer any of the times. She started becoming worried and was trying to convince my dad to turn around. He wasn't having it because we were almost to Florida, and he was determined to spend three full days alternating between golf and drinking beers in the pool.

When we stopped at a gas station, my mom went to a phone booth and called our neighbor. My dad and I stayed in the car and honked the horn about 40 times before an attendant came outside and told my dad to stop. My mom waited and waited for our neighbor to call back, and we could tell that what he told her wasn't good because she started pacing in the booth and then started crying, and she looked like she was going to have a meltdown.

The nurse who was supposed to be staying at our house stayed there for two nights. She threw a party on the third night. The neighbor told my mom that he thought the nurse was one of my older cousins or something because she had company coming and going all the days she was at our house. He said he heard a lot of noise, but he didn't want to call the police and start trouble. Our neighbor found my Grandma on the bathroom floor, barely conscious, and covered in her own excrement. He called 911, and medics said she was severely dehydrated. They took Grandma to the emergency room, and we headed back home right away.

My parents, of course, were beyond your typical angry. The nursing service apologized and offered a partial refund of our money, and then they said they were going to 'launch an investigation.' My mom said that wasn't good enough, and only when she threatened to sue did the nursing service say the 'nurse' they sent didn't have valid credentials. They routinely hired 'nurses' from newspaper ads for babysitters, saying that's essentially the type of care they offered. The nursing service told my mom that if she pursued legal action, she was going to make the 'nurse's' life hard, and that she should really consider that because it wasn't fair to the 'nurse.'

We eventually found out that my Grandma had fallen on the first night we were gone. The 'nurse' LEFT her there! My Grandma went without food or water for all that time, and she had no choice but to relieve herself as she lay on the floor. Grandma was in the hospital for weeks, suffering from a number of illnesses and injuries that stemmed from that incident.

And our house... Ooh, were my parents mad. The house was completely torn apart. I remember not being allowed to go in the kitchen or walk around the house barefoot for weeks because there was so much broken glass. In my room, all my posters were either torn off the walls or defaced. Someone had gone through my diary, a pre-teen's most sacred possession, and scribbled all over the entries. My goldfish, Rusty, was dead, and there were cigarette butts in his bowl. For some reason, my closet smelled like pee. It was nasty. We didn't have the money to hire a cleaning service (and by that time my mom was DONE with services, anyway), so a bunch of people from our neighbor's church came over a few weekends in a row, and they helped us either clean or replace things that were too damaged to be cleaned.

My mom and dad hired an attorney and discovered that this nursing service had conned others, so they joined a lawsuit. I don't think they ever saw a dime of their money, though. I don't think anyone in the lawsuit ever really got any answers. I know my parents notified law enforcement, and I'd like to be able to tell you that someone *at least* went to prison for this, but I don't remember my parents ever talking about it.

I think my mom has blamed herself all these years for what happened. Truthfully, there wasn't a lot she could have done, at least I don't think. Maybe she could have called the BBB (Better Business Bureau) to see if there had been complaints. Maybe she could have called a nursing home to see if they had some type of in-home service. I don't know.

I am not in nursing, so this isn't a story of why I joined the healthcare field. My boyfriend is studying to become an Anesthesiologist, so he's turned me on to your books. This is the only healthcare-related story that I think I have, and I didn't notice anyone had submitted something like this before, so I thought I'd share with your readers that one year a fake nurse almost let my Grandma die and ruined our family vacation.

-Initials and location withheld at request

All Fun and Games

Here are a few submissions that revolve around injuries sustained from toys or mishaps stemming from toys.

My grandson received a Wii console when the games were new to the market. He was attempting to teach me how to play the bowling game. I must have let the remote slip from my hand as I was following through, because boy, that remote flew up and hit me smack-dab in the mouth. I cracked my front tooth and had to see an emergency dentist.

-C.E.

Kansas

For Christmas, my mother-in-law bought the kids hoverboards. As expected, we experienced several bumped heads, broken lamps, and my eldest accidentally jerked forward and ran into the wall, leaving a hole in the plaster.

Enough was enough. I told the kids to put the boards on the chargers, and they could try again the next day, after we went out for knee pads and helmets. The kids complained, but they'd soon forgotten about the hoverboards and were then infatuated with video games. Bedtime came shortly after, and we all went to sleep.

I woke in the middle of the night because I was thirsty and also couldn't remember if I had switched the laundry. While I was approaching the laundry room, I smelled something burning. I followed the smell around the downstairs until I saw smoke coming from our enclosed back porch. One of the kids' hoverboard chargers had overheated and set the porch carpet on fire! Thankfully, I had a fire extinguisher in the garage.

To be on the safe side, I called the fire department and asked them to come out. I contacted the hoverboard company the next morning.

-B.N.
California

My kids and I were horsing around in the yard. After a while of them pestering me, I decided to take a turn on their generic Slip N Slide. I veered off course and hit a cement bird bath head-on. At first, I was too shocked to know that something was wrong. When I tried to get up, I felt the worst pain I've ever felt. I told one of my sons called 911. I sustained a neck fracture and was fitted with a Halo brace.

To be fair, the product came with a height and weight restrictions that I did not follow. Also, we had so much junk in the yard that someone was bound to get hurt. I'm just glad it was me, not the kids.

-B.B.

Location withheld at request

My daughter was crying because she shot herself in the face with her brother's Nerf gun, so I tried to make her stop crying by saying, "Look, it doesn't hurt."

I shot myself in the face and ended up in the ER with a corneal abrasion.

-F.T().
Wyoming

I threw my back out trying to hula hoop. That was a painful, embarrassing moment.

-K.H.
Utah

My husband promised he was going to do the dishes, but when I got home, I realized he hadn't. ALL our silverware was dirty. All of it. I don't know what my husband and three kids do when I'm not home, but I assume they have fancy dinners where they invite half the neighborhood, because it seems like a nightly thing where every single dish in the house is dirty.

Anyway, I wanted a hot roll with strawberry jam before I went to bed, so I thought I could get away with using a plastic serrated knife from my daughter's toy kitchen set. (She'd left the knife on the counter, so it's not like I went digging through her toy box.)

I was having difficulty getting the package of rolls open, so I tried using the plastic knife to cut the plastic. That worked. As I was trying to cut the roll in half, my hand slipped, and I cut my thumb open. I tried to bandage it, but there was just so much blood that I had to go back to work (I work in Respiratory), register as a patient in the ER, and get three stitches.

My husband never even knew I'd come home or left again until I told him about the mishap a few hours later, as he was getting up with the kids.

-A.B.
Oregon

Got the kids a good ol' fashioned tire swing, and I wanted to ensure I knotted the rope properly. I hopped up on the tire and the rope came undone from the tree branch immediately. I rode ass-up in the ambulance and was wheeled that way around the hospital for scans, only to learn I'd just suffered from 'intense' bruising.

-J.M.
South Carolina

Scary

We received an OD. This patient was delivered to us by an unknown person(s), and was essentially dumped in front of the ED. Witnesses claim the driver reached across the patient to open the passenger door, shoved the patient out of the vehicle, and sped off. Nobody managed to describe the driver or vehicle in detail, which does not surprise me. Had I witnessed the drop off, I am relatively positive I would also have been more concerned about the patient.

Most of the patient's veins were blown, making it increasingly difficult to do our jobs. The patient's extremities were covered in abscesses from drug abuse, and his/her appearance resembled something similar to a movie monster, due to the nature of his/her skin and overall condition. We stat paged Lab directly following our call to Respiratory. While we were waiting for both departments, the patient entered cardiac arrest.

Lab came in and during the commotion commented that one vein in the patient's arm felt blocked. I didn't know what she meant, exactly, as it could refer to a variety of complications. One of the doctors ordered us to start a line 'wherever we could,' and we'd figure everything else out later. We briefly contemplated starting a line in the patient's foot, as we felt we were running out of viable options. Luckily, Lab found a workable spot in the patient's neck that we'd overlooked.

We eventually discovered needles in the patient's arms and legs, ranging in length of flecks to inches, likely broken off during drug use.

I do not feel it would be appropriate to discuss the patient's outcome. The experience was one I will not soon forget.

-Initials and location withheld at request

Overheard by D.H. in Orgeon, while she was leaving for the day:

"Don't tell me you can't do it! I just watched a video where they did surgery on a grape!"

Stabbed in the...

One night, this gentleman calmly walked to my counter. I didn't notice a wobble or anything, and he didn't look ill, so I believed he was a visitor. Security was busy and I was taking an admit call from another facility, so I told the man if he was visiting, he needed to wait on the bench for someone to assist him.

He told me, "I can't sit."

I responded, "Sir, you need to wait until I can find someone to assist you."

He muttered something under his breath and walked away. I wasn't looking at him when he walked away.

A few minutes passed. I had to place the other facility on hold twice because patients had come in to be seen for non-critical injuries or cold symptoms. The visiting gentleman was standing near the entrance, facing me.

I ended my admit call and told the man, "I'm finding someone to help you now."

He thanked me and waited as I called around. I finally paged an orderly and informed the man someone was on the way.

When the orderly arrived, he asked the gentleman, "Where to, pal?"

"Uh, I don't know. Not surgery, I hope," the man replied.

The orderly nodded and asked, "If you don't know which floor the person you're visiting is on, we can ask this young lady to search the facility directory. If the patient is listed as accepting visitors, I can take you up there."

The man looked confused and said, "Oh, I'm not here to visit. I need to see a doctor."

At first, I was kind of mad and thought to myself, 'Well, why didn't you just tell me that? Duh.' But then I thought that I had not really given him a chance to tell me he was a patient.

I apologized to the orderly and asked the patient to come to the counter. I took his information. He was a new patient, so since the lobby was empty, I 'cheated' and gathered his details up front. This would save us both time in the long run, and it would basically allow the patient to leave as soon as he was discharged.

"And what brings you to the hospital?" I asked.

He told me, "This dude stabbed my ass."

"You were stabbed in the buttocks?" I asked.

He giggled and said, "I just call it the ass, but yeah."

I thought he was joking at first, and I was in a state of disbelief.

"Someone stabbed you in the butt?" I asked again.

He turned around. His jeans were saturated with blood. He pulled down his pants and boxers and showed me a gaping wound on his derriere. Just as he did this, another man was walking in. I recognized that man as a visitor to OB. He was on his cell phone and said loudly, "Oh, man, there's a guy standing in the ER with his junk hanging out."

"Okay," I said in a rush. "You can pull your pants up now."

The gentleman didn't pull his pants up. He went on to explain, "Well, that's why I couldn't sit. I wasn't trying to disrespect you. I just couldn't sit because I got stabbed in the ass. Is it bad? Does it look bad?"

"Sir," I said, as I picked up the phone to call a nurse, "please pull your pants up."

I don't know how many stitches the guy had to get, but I know that he screamed like a baby while he was getting them. As he was leaving, he told me the shot they gave him in the back hurt worse than the knife that had produced the wound. I don't know how he sustained the wound because the cops were outside and wanted to talk to him before he left hospital grounds.

That was the weirdest wound I've ever seen. I guess our hospital is boring.

-V.R.
Virginia

Recording

I work in EMS and wish to first and foremost warn that comments expressed in this submission are my own. I cannot and do not speak for my entire profession, but I believe what I wish to say is relatable to anyone in the first responder field.

I responded to a multi-vehicle MVA. One patient was extracted from a vehicle and CPR was started. Another patient was trapped in a second vehicle. We could not remove the patient, so one of us stayed with the patient and spoke to the patient while we awaited Fire.

A crowd had already gathered. One of our people asked the crowd to stay at a safe distance. We largely ignored the public because this is a common occurrence in EMS, at least in all the areas in which I have worked. If there are people nearby, we will have a crowd. It's unavoidable.

With curious crowds often follows cell phone recordings. For the sake of patient privacy, one of us (and in this case I mean EMS, LEO, Fire, etc.)

will attempt to reason with the bystander. We do not wish to see these recordings be uploaded to Facebook, especially before the patients are even loaded for transport. At particularly horrific scenes, our major concern regarding these recordings is that patients will be shown online, clearly deceased or in their last moments of life. This presents an issue of morality, for one, and we also don't want families to see their loved ones dead before someone has a chance to properly notify them. Many people seem to forget that while it is never 'easy' for a first responder to deliver news of a patient's passing to family members, we are often trained in this, at least somewhat.

Anyway, we noticed someone was recording as we were performing CPR, but we continued without giving the bystander attention. Fire came and extracted the patient in the other vehicle. We did everything we could for our first patient, but there was nothing more we could do. (Author's Note: Segments of this section have been omitted and edited with the reader's permission for clarification of the patient's status without submitting details that may identify the patient.)

We decided to move to assisting the patient from the other vehicle.

While we were working on the other patient, the bystander marched over to us and started accusing us of not giving the first patient enough medical intervention. This person snidely asked, "Excuse me, but I want to know why you stopped helping them."

We tried to move the bystander away from our patient and away from the scene in general, but the bystander began shouting about litigation and abuse of force. They were slapping us and saying that we were heartless because we just 'let' the patient die and we 'didn't care.' An LEO arrived moments later and attempted to reason with the bystander, but they were belligerent and violent. This behavior escalated and resulted in the bystander dropping his/her cell phone (which broke) and being placed under arrest.

This behavior sickens me. Like I said, I'm not the voice of paramedics everywhere, but I can tell you that I remember the face of every single patient who dies under my care or on my scene. Don't you dare walk up to a scene and tell me that I didn't do enough. Don't you dare try to flip it around and make it look like I favorited another patient. Don't come at me with no knowledge of this profession and tell me that I'm wrong because you saw an actor on TV do something different for a fake patient. This isn't TV. This is reality, and I worked hard to get where I am, and I work hard every single day to make sure that families can be reunited. I've held more hands than I can count. I've lied to people as they've laid dying on the side of the road by telling them it's going to be okay. Don't come up to me or anyone doing this job and accuse us of not caring.

I don't think we will see a decline in bystanders recording. I can even appreciate the fact that some recordings can be beneficial to the patient/subject and/or departments involved with the call. Recording just because you want to be internet famous is crossing the line. When we're on a call, we don't know what you're planning to do with that video, so excuse me if I'm angry that you're following my every movement. I can tell you that, personally, I'm never worried that I'm breaking protocol (in a way that is dangerous for the patient or my people). But it doesn't mean that I don't think that someone's not recording for that very purpose, of trying to catch me doing something wrong just so they can end my career.

I don't know what the world has become, I really don't. I'm sorry if any of this came off as trying to mandate what others are allowed to do. I just wish people would use some discretion when they're watching us, and never, ever, EVER approach a scene to interrupt patient care.

-W.D.
Location withheld at request

One of my coworkers went to the news with something illegal she'd seen happen in our ER. She only did this because the hospital swept the incident under the rug. The hospital found out and found a reason to fire her that had nothing to do with going to the news station. My coworker never fought it because she didn't really care if she was fired from this crappy place. She said she went to a lawyer, though, when one of our bosses threatened her and said if she talked to the media again the hospital would sue.

What does it say about your business if you care more about people finding out than you care about making sure these things don't happen?

-L.F.
Indiana

We were pleasantly surprised to see a mom and her daughter standing outside the ER as we went off shift at 07:00. They had set up a table and were selling Girl Scout cookies to nurses as we came on and off shift.

I don't know whose idea that was, but it was a genius one.

I heard security made them leave. I bet that little girl made a killing because I know I bought eight boxes.

-I.H.
Vermont

PTO

With 20 minutes left until I was scheduled for a 14-hour shift, I went to light a cigarette. (It's a bad habit, I know.) I couldn't find my lighter, so I turned on one of my stove's burners and leaned in to get a light.

I never stopped to think about the new products I'd put in my hair: a light olive oil leave-in mask, followed by hair spray.

I realized right away that my hair was on fire, but it took me a moment to react. Luckily, I was able to pat out the flames.

I investigated the damage in the mirror. My hair was originally shoulder-length and curly. Following the incident, one side of my hair was that long, but on the side that caught fire, my hair ended at the center of my ear. My neck was a little red, but thankfully the flames just went after the product in my hair.

Mortified, I called work and gave Charge the rundown. She said she felt bad for me, but we were already short, and nobody could stay over. I even asked if I could work a partial shift, thinking I could just wear a cap over my head or something. She said no and said that if I felt I was in such need of a night off, I needed to register as a patient, because that was the only way I'd be excused from work. I asked to speak Unit Manager because I felt this was unfair.

When I spoke to our Unit Manager, I explained that I had more than 400 hours of PTO saved up. I explained the situation and requested the night off. She denied my request and said that she was not confident that she would have even accepted my request if I had called earlier because my 'first duty' should be to the hospital.

I was too afraid to stand up for myself, so I went to work…right after I took a pair of scissors and cut off the other side of my hair. I was in tears all night. I understand the problem with me giving 20 minutes of notice to call in, but I don't understand why they couldn't work with me. And what would they have done if I had died on my way to work, or if one of my coworkers had gotten ill? I never did file a complaint with management because I could see that my version of an emergency was not their version of one.

A few months later, I learned management had canceled my upcoming PTO. I had already gotten a week off approved. My sister was being induced and her husband passed shortly after they learned they were pregnant, so I wanted to be with her during the birth. When I confronted management about this, I was told the time I'd requested off coincided with hospital training that had not even been scheduled when I put in my request, and again, my priority should be work.

I went back to my desk, typed up my notice, and turned it in a few moments later. Thankfully, that hospital pays out PTO when you leave your position. It was not ideal because I had to pay taxes on that large payout. However, it was still enough that I could stay with my sister.

Maybe that hospital wouldn't be consistently short-staffed if they could appreciate the staff they do have. I'm much happier at my new job…And they don't restrict PTO!

-H.H.
Indiana

First Date

So, my partner and I were dispatched to a report of a hit and run. Our patient had been cycling when he was hit by a motorist. The patient's girlfriend was ridiculously loud and annoying, especially because the patient was not that bad off.

While we were assessing the patient and running down our on-site checklist, the patient's girlfriend went between sobbing loudly and then behaving erratically. At one point, she even asked with a pout, "Why is nobody paying attention to me?"

The patient was visibly upset by his girlfriend's behavior. I asked one of the officers on scene, "Can you take our patient's girlfriend over there for a minute? I need to ask him some personal questions."

"She's not my girlfriend," the patient blurted out, waving his hands like 'no way.'

At the same time, the female said, "You can ask me personal questions. Hey, do you want to see something cool?"

She then lifted her leg and stuck it behind her head while she was standing.

(Don't worry, she was wearing leggings.)

None of us knew what to say. We were just like, "Uh, okay."

A female officer walked the woman away from the scene. I heard her ask, "Ma'am, have you consumed any drugs or alcohol today?"

The female laughed and said, "Nope! I'm just peppy!"

I asked our patient, "So, uh, not your girlfriend?"

He said, "That was hot, but she's insane."

He explained that the two met on some dating website and were on their first date. It was the first time I'd ever heard someone tell me they were glad they were hit by a car. He said the woman had started talking about marrying him 10 minutes after they met in person, and he thought he could tolerate her long enough to finish their bike ride and then tell her they weren't compatible.

The patient was okay, but he requested medical transport anyway because his bike was too damaged to ride home, and he told my partner and me that he wanted to get away from his date as fast as possible. Apparently, their date was so bad that he was willing to risk a hefty medical transport bill. We kind of talked to the other officer on scene while the one officer was trying to keep the patient's date entertained. The cop said he'd tell the patient he needed him to come to the station to answer some questions, and he and his partner would give the guy a ride home.

The last time I looked over, the patient's date was trying to do cartwheels and kept running up to random people walking and jogging through the park, trying to get their attention.

-G.T.
Illinois

I scheduled a patient with our clinic for a complaint of 'just feeling sick.'

Our N.P. asked me to call the police about 10 minutes after she entered the exam room to meet the patient.

This man stated he healthy. His reason for the visit? He was trying to buy medication (specifically antibiotics and opioids) in bulk under the table from our clinic. He was convinced the world was about to end. As officers were escorting him out, the man was screaming that we would all be sorry when he was the 'King of the New World.'

I was scared he'd come back, but we haven't seen him since.

-Initials and location withheld at request

I answered an anonymous call to our non-emergency line one night.

The female asked, "Hey, if I break into the zoo after hours, will I go to prison?"

I said, "Depending on your criminal history, it's a possibility. I wouldn't recommend doing that."

Before I could say anything else, she said, "Okay, thanks," and hung up.

We didn't receive any calls regarding a break-in at the zoo that night, so I am assuming she took my advice.

-E.B.
Ohio

Premium

I had been at the hospital nearly every single hour of the day for 16 days straight. I forced myself to take a late-night break from the hospital at the recommendation of my daughter's wonderful nurses.

When I was coming back from getting decaf coffee, I'd realized I'd forgotten the special badge they'd given me to open the doors to the unit. I had to go to the ER desk and request someone either call for a nurse to escort me or see if a security officer could give me a badge.

I showed the officer my driver's license and he said he'd have to call up to make sure I was on the visitor's sheet.

He asked, "You said your baby is upstairs?"

I nodded and said, "Yes. She's a preemie. I just needed a break."

The clerk at the desk must not have understood what that meant because she scoffed and said, "Your kid is no better than anyone else's. You have some nerve walking around here, talking about having a premium baby. There's no such thing as a premium baby. They're all the same."

I just kind of looked at her because that's such a stupid statement for anyone to make.

She bugged her eyes at me and asked, "What? Do you have a problem?"

The thing is, I work in a hospital. I know the difference between losing your temper or responding to a rude person versus being hostile when nothing's been directed towards you. I was too tired to argue with anyone, and it seemed so silly to engage, anyway.

I don't know what her problem was, but I mentioned the incident to a nurse once I was back with my daughter.

-R.H.
Ohio

We had a woman come to our front desk and complain, "There's some kind of demonic ritual going on outside."

When I went to the parking lot to investigate, a group of heavily tattooed, leather-clad bikers had joined in a circle and were holding hands while they prayed (what I would consider a traditional non-Satanic prayer) for their friend, who had been admitted for cardiac complications.

I can only assume the woman had misjudged the group by their appearance. They never gave us any trouble, so I didn't have any complaints.

-O.W.
Florida

That's Offensive!

We were talking about going out after work. I made the comment, "I don't like Mexican food. Most of it's too spicy."

I have severe Crohn's, so I limit myself to what others call 'boring' foods. My flare-ups have landed me in the hospital several times, including when I've been on vacation. I have to choose my meals wisely, or I'm going to be miserable.

A patient overheard me and filed a complaint with the hospital because my statement was 'offensive.'

My coworkers had to write statements that we were talking about FOOD and that I was NOT badmouthing an ethnicity, but simply expressing my personal preferences over where we were going to meet for supper.

Thankfully, I didn't get in any trouble, but we were all given a verbal warning (a reminder, really) to keep our discussions work-related because patients can hear us at all times and may find it unprofessional that we get hungry. (I'm being sarcastic, so please translate that into the text.)

What's this world coming to?!

-D.E.
California

That's Not How Those Work

My patient registered and was in the waiting room. I asked the registration clerk, "What kind of medication problem? Did he tell you what was going on?"

The clerk shrugged and replied, "I don't really know. He said he bought some pills at Walgreens and they weren't working right."

My mind went to 'allergic reaction.'

I called the patient back and triaged him. I then addressed his chief complaint and asked, "Sir, what kind of problem are you having with your medication?"

This man gave me his entire life story, starting from birth. I mean that literally. When I tried to interrupt him, he'd ignore me and continue his story.

Eleven years and 47,000 shifts later, he got around to detailing to his trip to the store. He'd had diarrhea after eating too much pie, and he bought some OTC anti-diarrheal medicine. He handed me a box of pills.

"And it's just not working," he said.

"So, you still have some diarrhea?" I asked.

He nodded and said, "But it's not just that. I've been trying to get it all out of there, but I just can't. Some of them have broken up and are stuck."

"What are stuck?" I asked.

"Those," he said, nodding to the package I'd placed on my rolling desk.

'Oh, tell me he didn't,' I thought.

"Where are they stuck?" I asked.

He shrugged and said, "You know, where the BM comes out."

I picked up the box and asked, "You inserted this medication rectally?"

He nodded.

"Sir," I explained, "this medication says to take orally."

He exclaimed, "You mean I was 'sposta swallow them?"

I gulped and nodded.

"Well, I'll be a son of a bitch," the guy muttered.

He shook his head while I sat in silence. Then he laughed and asked, "Think I can get some suppositories? Those suckers always stop me right up."

I chuckled and told the patient, "Let's take you to a room, and we'll see what we can do."

-M.N.
Alabama

Love and Marriage

I returned from escorting my patient to the restroom and noticed how my coworkers were behaving oddly. A code had come in, so I thought maybe something was going on. I didn't know for sure. I just helped my patient back to bed, and I went to the nurses' station.

Charge asked me to take my break early, which is really what got the bells ringing in my head. I thought I was going to be fired. I didn't do anything wrong (to my knowledge), but I have anxiety, so I always see red flags.

I was uneasy, but I accepted her order. I just had to grab my water bottle from my desk, and I relayed that to her. She was in the middle of a sentence, trying to tell me not to look at my computer monitor, when I noticed my husband's name on the screen.

Naturally, I panicked. I may have been screaming, I'm honestly not sure. My brain put the code and my husband's name together before I could even read the chief complaint on the screen.

My coworkers tried to calm me down, but I sprinted towards the room where the response team and my coworkers were performing compressions on a motionless male patient.

Someone screamed at me, "What are you doing?" as I tried to push everyone out of the way.

My heart was racing. I was crying. My chest hurt, and I couldn't breathe. I felt like I'd just run a one-minute mile with a killer bear on my heels.

Charge and an orderly yanked me out of the room and told me to calm down.

I screamed, "Tell me where my f*cking husband is!"

Charge said, "You need to calm down. Go take your break, and we'll talk later."

I'm friends with her outside of work. I knew her before I started at this ER. Ordinarily, under almost any other circumstance, I would have trusted her. But something didn't feel right.

Just a few seconds later, a tech stuck his head out from a room and said, "Hey, your husband's in here. He said to tell you…"

The tech blushed and looked around before continuing, "I can't say what he said. But he said you can come in."

I had snot streaming down my face when I entered my husband's room. He was sitting on the edge of the bed, holding a towel over his arm.

"I told him to tell you to stop [freaking] screaming at everyone and just come in here," he said to me.

I don't think I've ever been more relieved to see my husband. I grabbed about 32 tissues from the box on the counter to wipe my face, and then my brain went into RN mode.

I demanded he tell me why he was in the ER and told him to show me his arm.

He told me he didn't want me to know he was a patient, but he said, "I messed up bad."

I groaned because he has a history of injuries sustained while performing stupid activities. He's always been a bit of an Evel Knievel mixed with the guys from Dumb and Dumber.

When he lifted the towel, there was a gash that went from his elbow to his wrist.

I gasped and asked, "How did you do that?"

"You don't want to know," he told me.

I inspected the wound and noticed there were knotted fibers present.

"What did you do?" I demanded, pointing to the blue string.

"I'd rather tell you how I cut my arm," he said.

I sighed.

He told me he was trying to hang a decorative metal sun with a mirror in its center that I'd been 'nagging' him to hang for two years. First of all, I wouldn't have to 'nag' if we could have the mirror hanged instead of buying it and leaving it in the closet. Secondly, I don't know that asking him every three months for a year and a half would be considered 'nagging.' But, apparently, he'd gotten around to hanging the piece, so he brought in the ladder from the garage. The ladder didn't reach, so get this.

My husband pulled an armchair over to the wall, put the ladder on the armchair, and then he said he climbed and 'just kept hoping' it didn't fall.

Of course, the chair scooted away from the wall, causing the ladder to fall…while my husband was on it. He landed on the sun he'd been holding. One of the sun's rays sliced his arm open.

"I'm gonna clean up the mess before you get home," he assured me.

"But what's all that stuff in the cut?" I asked him.

"You don't want to know," he said again.

I gave him 'the look,' so he confessed that he tried to sew the wound with a handheld sewing machine-like device I'd purchased to patch up my jeans. That was the worst $20 I'd ever spent, so I threw it in the junk room and forgotten about it.

"You didn't!" I hissed.

He glanced down and said, "Well, it didn't work."

I love my husband, but sometimes I wonder about his thought process.

My husband ended up getting 27 sutures, and I was pulled aside after he was discharged and scolded on my behavior. I apologized and said I'd panicked. Charge said she had wanted me to go on break because she tried to follow hospital policy. My husband said no to our facility directory and asked that I not be notified that he was in the ER. I don't know what he would've done if I'd been sitting at my computer when he came in, but I'm guessing that he didn't see me when my coworker brought him back, so he figured he'd try to be in and out without me ever noticing that he was there. I don't know how he expected to explain away the bills or the broken sun mirror or, you know, the fact that he'd have 27 sutures in his arm.

-J.L.
Arkansas

Obscene

I work in Admitting and have to share something mindboggling that I witnessed. I think this will be something I remember for the rest of my life.

My coworker registered a patient to be seen in our ED. The patient is well-known to our hospital. He's a polite gentleman, very quiet and never one to cause a scene. This gentleman is an amputee. He uses a wheelchair for mobility. He owns prosthetics, but he does not prefer to use them.

This gentleman was patiently waiting in the waiting area for his turn. A family walked in and the mother of three demanded all five members of her family be seen for exposure to influenza. I was angry right off the bat because I had been nothing but nice to this woman, her husband, and her bratty kids. It was unnecessary for her to treat me so disrespectfully. When I tried to gather any information that pertained to her family's primary care physicians, she rolled her eyes and told me,

"You're just a registration clerk. You only need to know what I tell you." I felt that was uncalled for.

I asked the family to wait in the waiting room and advised the woman that I would estimate the wait time to be at least 30 minutes. I said the nurses would likely place each adult in a separate room and split the kids between the two rooms.

The woman said, "Well, you don't really *know* they'll do that, do you?"

I said, "No, but that's what they usually do when families come in to be seen."

She said, "If you don't *know,* then you should just keep your mouth shut."

I told her to go to the waiting room and wait to be called. She was complaining loudly as she walked away that she was going to report me. At that point, I couldn't care less if she reported me.

Roughly two minutes after the family went to the waiting room, the woman came marching back to my work area.

I wanted to say, "Oh great, you're already back to bitch some more," but I didn't.

She said, "You need to do something about this."

"About what?" I asked.

"You shouldn't put people like that where normal people go to wait."

I didn't know what she was talking about because there were not many people left in the waiting room, and I didn't think any in the room had acted strangely when I'd seen them.

"Did someone do something?" I asked.

She told me to stop acting like I didn't know what was wrong.

I said, "I can't help you if I don't know what your problem is."

She screamed, "I am not the one with a problem! You people are sick for letting someone like that wait where normal people are sitting."

"Who are you talking about?" I asked, sighing heavily.

"That freak with no legs!" she shouted.

"Ma'am," I said sharply, "please don't call anyone names."

"I can say what I damn-well want to," she shouted. "You need to get that freak out of there. He's scaring my kids."

I glanced over to the waiting area. Nobody seemed to be exhibiting signs of distress.

"Did that gentleman say or do something that upset you?" I asked.

"He doesn't have any legs," the woman growled.

"Ma'am," I said, "if he's not said or done something wrong, I can't ask him to leave the waiting room."

The woman started calling me names and grew louder by the second.

Finally, I picked up the phone and called for help.

The woman shouted at me, "You know what? Never mind. I'm taking my kids out of this shit hospital. I'm telling everyone on Facebook about this."

"About how you're freaking out about a disabled veteran?" I asked angrily.

"I shouldn't have to see freaks like that," the woman screamed. "I don't even know why he thought it would be okay to leave his house like that. Nobody else should have to be forced to see someone like that."

I lost my temper and said, "Funny, because I feel the same way about seeing someone like you in public."

I didn't mean this as an attack on her physical features, but more about her behavior.

She then said I was discriminating against her and her family by taking a 'freak's' side.

The woman stomped back to the waiting room and yelled, "Come on. We're leaving."

Her husband and children got up from their seats and put their jackets back on.

You'd think the woman would stop there, but she didn't. She started yelling at the patient, screaming about how he was 'gross' and an 'abomination.' She was too stupid to know how to pronounce the word 'abomination,' so sometimes it'd come out as 'Obama's nation' or 'a bomb action.'

The patient's husband acted like he'd seen this happen a million times before, so he wasn't affected at all. I bet the woman does this kind of stuff all the time, so her husband is probably used to it.

We don't have security guards, so I had to wait until two techs could make it to the ER from upstairs. They had to basically step between the woman and the patient and keep walking toward the woman until she backed out of the ER.

Even though I really had nothing to apologize for, I went to the waiting room and apologized to the patient for how he was treated by the woman and her family. I told him I was sorry that I couldn't get help down to the waiting room quicker than I did, and that I was sorry that he had to experience that. He thanked me and said it didn't bother him because he was used to dealing with ignorant people.

I never saw the woman or her family again. If we're being honest here, I hope I never see her again. I asked the patient if I could share this story, and he said it was okay. He said anything that brings awareness to how disabled veterans are treated is important to him.

-C.P.
Louisiana

Irritating Patient

A woman walked in the ER and complained into her cell phone as she waited in line. She was incredibly rude and the observations she was making about others ahead of her were insulting. Of course, she used the line, "I thought this was the emergency room" about 900 times in the five minutes it took me to register and/or assist the people in front of her.

When it came time for me to help the woman, she made me wait for her to finish her conversation. I tapped on a sign that we have taped to the front desk, which reads, "PLEASE, NO CELL PHONE USAGE AT TIME OF REGISTRATION."

The woman rolled her eyes and said, "I don't give a shit about your stupid sign. You work for me."

I wanted to strangle her right then and there, but management frowns upon staff attacking patients.

When I became fed up of the woman talking smack about me while she stood right in front of me, holding up the line, I stood up and called the next person to the counter.

The woman on the phone told the person she was speaking with that she'd call them back, and then she told the person I'd called to the front to 'learn his place.' She went on to tear me a new one. I informed her that I can't put my job on hold just because she was taking a phone call. She started cussing me again.

"Do you need to be seen for medical treatment?" I interrupted. This brought on a lecture about interrupting people.

The patients behind the woman were growing just as irritated as I was.

Finally, the woman told me that yes, she did need to be seen. Her chief complaint isn't important to add, but she said she expected to be in and out in 'five or ten minutes.' I just kind of stared at her and said I hadn't even seen *wait* times that short for three weeks. She cussed me again.

I am allowed to ask patients to stop cursing at me, but I'm not allowed to ask them to leave. I have to register them no matter what. I can call security, and they can ask the patient to stop cursing at me, but they can't ask the patient to leave. It's really screwed up because this woman was hateful from the start and basically, there was nothing anyone could do about it. I make $9 an hour to basically be a verbal punching bag for people, and it sucks. You can tell me to get another job all you want, but someone else will have to take my place, and the point is, is that nobody should be subjected to being treated this way. Employers need to do more to take care of their employees. I don't care if I make $9 or $20 an hour. I shouldn't have to tolerate someone calling me racist names or cussing me because they have to wait five minutes in line. (AMEN!)

It took about four minutes to register the patient because when I'd ask her anything, she'd demand, "Why the hell do you need to know that?" or she'd tell me, "That's none of your f*cking business."

She vehemently refused to give me her driver's license, but then she didn't want to give me her name or date of birth because, "One of these assholes is gonna steal my identity."

"Ma'am," I said, "I need to know your information so I can get you in the system."

She finally spelled out her name for me. JAYNE SMYTH.

I confirmed this spelling THREE times. THREE. I had witnesses.

When I completed registration, I politely asked the patient to take a seat in the waiting room and someone would call her as soon as possible. I looked at my Tracking Board and noted that she was the third or fourth patient waiting for triage, so I'd estimate her wait time between 20 and 40 minutes, give or take (based on the seriousness of the complaints ahead of hers). She cussed me again but went to the waiting room.

They must've revved the engines in the back because three nurses came out at once to call patients. The rude patient I'd just sent to the waiting room was called back fewer than five minutes after I'd asked her to wait.

She was complaining the entire time she was walking with the nurse because I had 'lied' to her about how long it was going to take, and she had really wanted to finish watching the news segment that was on the waiting room television.

In my mind I groaned and thought, "You've got to be freaking kidding me." I hated this woman so much already.

Another patient came in, and his situation is what the ER is for. Just as I was reaching for the phone to call for help, it rang.

"Hey," I said as soon as I picked up the receiver, "I need help right now."

The nurse on the other end said, "Well, first I need you to change a patient's name. You spelled it wrong, and she's taking it out on me."

"Really need help," I repeated. "This guy looks like he's vomiting feces and blood at the same time."

"I'll send someone up. But I need you to change this patient's name. She's impossible to deal with, and I want her out of here ASAP."

I was trying to give the vomiting patient an emesis bag while remaining on the line with the nurse, but I must have stretched the cord too far because all I heard was silence. I was dodging pools of blood-tinged oatmealish liquid that smelled like bowel movements…At least I was until the patient vomited on my shoes.

I thought I was going to vomit, too, but I didn't. Two nurses kind of bumped me out of the way as they hurried to get the patient into a wheelchair.

One of the nurses said something like, "Yeah, there's no way this can't be an obstruction."

She told me to stat page janitorial services and start rerouting traffic to an entrance down the corridor. It was inconvenient, but it kept traffic from the vile scene in front of the ER doors.

"Why is my patient's name not changed in the computer?" the nurse from the back shouted, as she came rushing to the front.

She stopped right behind me, covered her nose with her hand, and then looked at my shoes. She said, "Oh my God! Someone vomited this all up?"

I have been the only one on shift when we've had possible active shooter scenarios. I've been on shift when there were brawls going on in the triage room (and lobby…and waiting room…and corridor). I've been physically attacked by patients. I even had a jail clearance pee on me once. But this was just too much.

I started sobbing. People who were waiting to be registered, who'd witnessed all the vomiting go down, tried consoling me. The nurse behind me guided me to my work area and used a towel to help me take off my shoes. Then she brought me surgical booties and a biohazard bag. She called the Unit Clerk up front to register patients.

I heard the first rude patient shouting from the back. The nurse who was trying to calm me down sighed and said, "I can't stand that woman. You messed up her name, so I really need that fixed so she can go home."

I sniffled and said, "I didn't mess up her name."

The nurse became frustrated, mostly out of stress I think, and showed me the patient's driver's license. The nurse said, "She said that she gave you her license and you still spelled her name wrong."

"She did not!" I shouted. "She refused to give me her license, and then I double checked the spelling SHE gave me THREE times!"

"Okay, okay," the nurse said. "Try to calm down."

"I hate that woman!" I screamed.

I don't care if it was unprofessional, and I don't care if anyone heard me. I was in 100% total meltdown mode.

The Unit Clerk only had the ability to register patients, not edit their information. I had to log on the triage nurse's laptop and change the patient's name from JAYNE SMYTH to JANE SMITH.

I ended up calling my mom to bring me another pair of shoes. My old shoes smelled so bad and were stained even after I washed them that I just threw them in the garbage.

-K.L.
New Jersey

That's Not Funny!

We have a wall near our work station, where we tape up cute medical-related comics we find online, in newspapers, or in medical quarterlies some of have subscriptions to. Well, we HAD a wall.

A patient's wife was leaning over our desk area to read the comics. She approached me and said, "You need to get that thing off the wall before I turn you guys in."

"Huh?" I asked.

She pointed to the wall and said, "That one, with the gown. Take it down now, or I'm turning you in."

I looked at the wall until I found the comic that so deeply bothered her. It was a silly drawing of a man wearing a hospital gown. He was sitting on the bed. All you could see was the patient's back. There was a nurse or doctor entering the room, and they were saying something like, "You put the gown on backwards!"

I think the point was to infer the patient's genitalia were exposed.

"This one?" I asked the patient's wife.

"Yes," she huffed. "It's not funny."

"I'm sorry," I said, "but I don't think there's anything offensive about this."

"I *just* told you that it's NOT funny. Take it down, or I'm turning you in."

I don't know why I became so enraged by this. I suppose I could have removed the comic, just to avoid the woman's additional complaints.

Instead I said, "It's not funny to *you*, but other people think it's funny."

She argued, "I don't care what other people think. It's not funny. Take it down now, or I'm turning you in."

This woman seemed to hold the belief that the louder she raised her voice, the more serious I would take her complaint.

I shrugged and said, "Then you'll have to turn me in."

I went back to my charting and referred the woman to her husband's nurse when she had anything else to say. I was done with a capital D.

The very next night, I came to work to see every single comic had been removed from the wall. There was a piece of paper taped there that instructed us to check our emails.

The patient's wife complained that the comic made light of people with intellectual disabilities, and that she found this comic to be the most offensive on the wall. She complained about other comics and threatened to 'make a stink' about it to 'everyone' she knew. To avoid bad press and appease the woman, administration decided it would be best that we take the comics down. We are not allowed to post anything that does not directly relate to patient care in our work area now. (We aren't even allowed to tape the carry-in sign up sheet on the wall. When I asked the House Super about it, I was told that administration was afraid that someone would complain that we were not focused on patient care. Uh, what? Sure, let's tape it in the break room that the vast majority of employees never enter because we're too busy to ever have a break.)

First off, NONE of those comics were what anyone in his or her right mind would consider offensive, but even if they were, does that mean that what you find offensive, I must also? Thank

God she didn't see the dirty comics we kept in the breakroom (not dirty as in sexual harassment, but dirty as in not needing to post a picture of a chicken undergoing plastic surgery with frozen chicken breasts purchased from the supermarket).

We moved the comic wall to the breakroom, but it doesn't feel the same. We used those comics to make time pass a little bit faster, to liven up the place just a bit. It's not like we were spending hours in front of the comics. We usually checked it while we were washing up or something.

Just wanted to say, "Thanks" to the woman who had a stick up her ass. I'm sure she's off forming a local branch of the thought police as I type this.

-T.A.
Oregon

Couldn't Be That Bad

On a busy overnight shift—one when I'd forgotten my lunch at home—I went digging through the break room fridge. I couldn't find anything in there, unless you counted 800 bottles of ranch dressing, half-empty bottles of water, and a bunch of empty Tupperware. I moved on to the cabinets and the contents looked pretty much the same. I was about to give up, but then I saw a box of oatmeal at the back. Wooh!

The box contained multiple packets of flavors, like apple cinnamon, plain, and strawberry. I like the apple kind, so I used hot water from the coffee machine and made myself a bowl of oatmeal.

As I was walking through the ER with my oatmeal, a few nurses asked what I had. "Oatmeal," I replied. "There's a whole box back there."

The nurses head that direction.

When I went back to wash my bowl, the box was empty. We'd gone through 16 packets of oatmeal in about 10 minutes.

About an hour later, a nurse came to the front and asked, "You know that oatmeal we ate?"

"Uh-huh," I mindlessly answered, as I was scrolling through Facebook.

"It expired six years ago."

None of us ended up getting sick, so that was a plus.

That's the story about the night we ate six-year-old oatmeal.

-P.S.
Michigan

A Message to Readers

I have been corresponding with many readers via social media, and I love it. I wanted to touch base with everyone and thank you. I'm grateful to have your support! I'm first going to address formatting changes, and then I will address a few messages and/or reviews I've received from readers.

Every now and then, I receive messages and/or reviews from readers put off by the series' formatting and repetitious nature. To be honest, I even become overwhelmed with the content at times. There's not much I can do regarding the repetitious nature of the content. If you work in the healthcare field (or any field, really), you'll find similarities in most stories long-term. I have been mindful of using too many (for example) submissions about assaults if the previous book covered several similar submissions.

As far as formatting is concerned, I've thought the formatting I've been using fit the overall theme of both series, but I HAVE listened, and I'm sure you've noticed this book has a *slightly* different format. It can be good to change things up. I HAVE NOT changed font size/spacing of the submissions, as this is key praise from readers suffering from failing eyesight or readers who just need a break from default settings. If this proves to be something most of you hate, I'll flip it back. Because these books are compilations of stories with various themes, I feel I'm limited on formatting options.

I am open to hearing any suggestions from YOU, the readers. I read most of these reviews/messages as constructive criticism and understand we all have different preferences. However, it's important to me that YOU are also satisfied. So, if anyone has suggestions, I'm always open to them.

Through some feedback, I'm learning I can't make everyone happy, and I understand that. Some people complain just to complain, and nothing will ever be good enough for them. I also understand that. I've made some mistakes with both series, and I own up to them. But, if there's something you think this series needs (besides an editor—ha ha—I know, I overlook things at times), I'm all ears.

Someone brought up the possibility of a fraudulent submission that was printed in a previous edition. Apparently, the reader included a statement regarding the Uber ride service, but the organization would not have been in service at the time the story occurred. I addressed the reader who brought this to my attention by replying to a review, but I want to include it in this section, as not everyone receives notifications that I've replied. Also, this is good information to get out there for everyone to see.

There are times it's obvious that a submission has been stolen from an internet joke or contains highly questionable content, and I do my best to weed those out of the running as book content. I've even received submissions that were pulled directly from my first series and submitted as the person's firsthand account, which was obvious because I'd recognize those stories immediately, as they happened to me (and one poor person didn't even bother to alter the story before sending it, so he/she copy/pasted my own words and tried to pass them off as his/her own, LOL). Admittedly, however, I'm probably sometimes guilty of overlooking the details of submissions because I'm too focused on the juicy details. That's a major error on my part.

With the submission in question, I had/have no reason to doubt it. Submissions often bounce around and stories are told out of chronological order and usually come with side stories/details that never make it to the final product. I'd like to give the reader the benefit of the doubt and believe Uber was used as a replacement word for a local ride service or perhaps is now synonymous to the reader as a taxi at the time the story occurred, just like [the person who brought this to my attention] suggested. I suppose it's entirely possible that this was a fabrication, but then again, I'd have to go back through every accepted piece and question its validity. I usually have email/message conversations with readers during the submission and acceptance process, and most people give detailed information (that never makes it to books) supporting their submissions. There are times that readers include detailed information regarding medications, treatments, injuries, and more that never make it to the end for one of two reasons: 1.) the information could potentially identify the patient and/or reader (even with submissions edited for other potential markers) , or 2.) the information is far too detailed to keep the books simple and fun for both first responders and also readers with little to no healthcare knowledge. This is why you almost never see dosages and specific medications, or procedures mentioned in either series. I usually will place 'blanket' terms in place of specifics because it's enough to share the experience but not compromise privacy and/or clutter the piece.

As far as I'm aware, this is the first time this issue has popped up (where it hasn't been caught in the acceptance process), and hopefully I'll do a better job of following the story prior to/during the acceptance process and paying attention when I'm editing. Especially in the Small-Town series, I took the cake on typos and screw ups (can't tell you how many times I've had to pull a book to add page numbers), so I'm more than willing to say this could have been an oversight on my end as far as letting one sneak by me.

With that being said, I whole-heartedly do not believe the reader intentionally included inaccurate information. If that occurred, then it's my own fault for not reviewing the submission in depth.

On another topic, a reader wrote:

"I recall reading in one of your earlier books something about failed suicide attempts. At the time, I was so upset that I put down the book and didn't touch it for months. I vowed to never read another one of your books. That passage seemed cold for not only someone employed by the healthcare system, but also for a human being. I still believe that your words could stand editing for clarity and compassion. The way you spoke about that topic was disturbing."

It is never my intention to alienate readers. My delivery does sometimes come off abrasively (so much so that the overall message is lost in the tone), but I do believe in extending compassion to everyone. Unfortunately, I have a bad habit of putting my foot in my mouth or not addressing topics sensitively or coming off as 'matter of fact.' I've come off pompous before (especially in the first book—I think it came off more of a bad attitude than humor, and I regret not going a different direction), and for that I apologize. Opinions can change, and I am always trying to grow as a person to have an open mind and see things from all sides. My opinion on this matter specifically does not only come from previously working in healthcare, but also from occurrences in my personal life that I may or may not address another time. Overall, I very much believe that we have a lack of resources available for mental health, and that we need to reduce the stigma associated with mental health issues.

You guys have been great, and I can't thank you enough. If you have questions or concerns, feel free to reach out to me. I do my best to respond to all messages in a timely manner.

Have a great day, guys!

Check me out on Twitter!
https://twitter.com/AuthorKerryHamm

You can also find me on Facebook, by searching for 'Author Kerry Hamm.'

www.ingramcontent.com/pod-product-compliance
Lightning Source LLC
Chambersburg PA
CBHW030612220526
45463CB00004B/1263